The Happy Healthy Plant-Based Cookbook

75+

Colorful Recipes to
Nourish Your Whole Body,
Feed Your Family &
Have Fun Along the Way

Dusty & Erin
Stanczyk

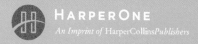

HarperOne
An Imprint of HarperCollinsPublishers

The Happy Healthy Plant-Based Cook-Book

FIRST EDITION

Designed by Bonni Leon-Berman
Photos by Erin Stanczyk, Dusty Stanczyk, Ariel Panowicz, Mirando Rossi, and Devon Stanczyk

Library of Congress Cataloging-in-Publication Data has been applied for.

ISBN 978-0-06-327117-3

24 25 26 27 28 LBC 5 4 3 2 1

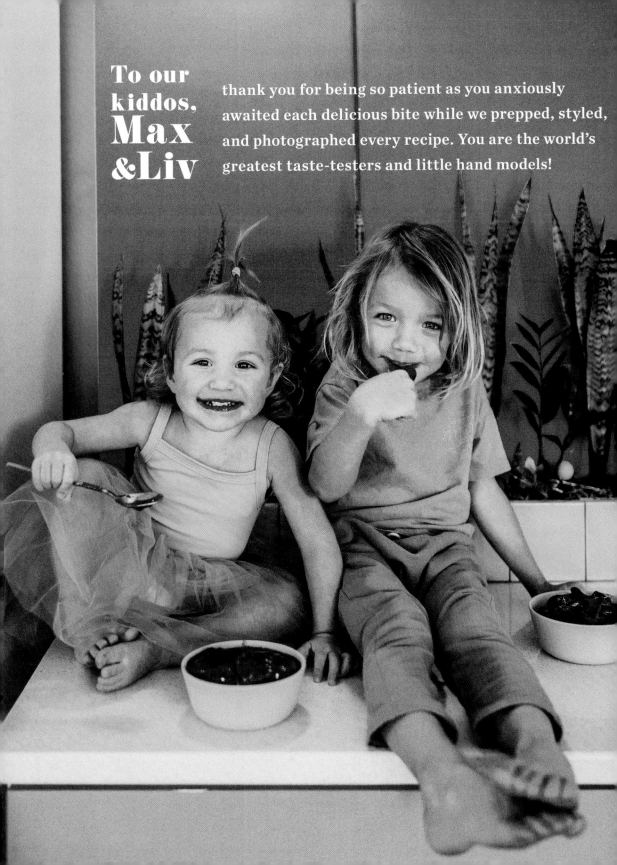

To our kiddos, Max &Liv

thank you for being so patient as you anxiously awaited each delicious bite while we prepped, styled, and photographed every recipe. You are the world's greatest taste-testers and little hand models!

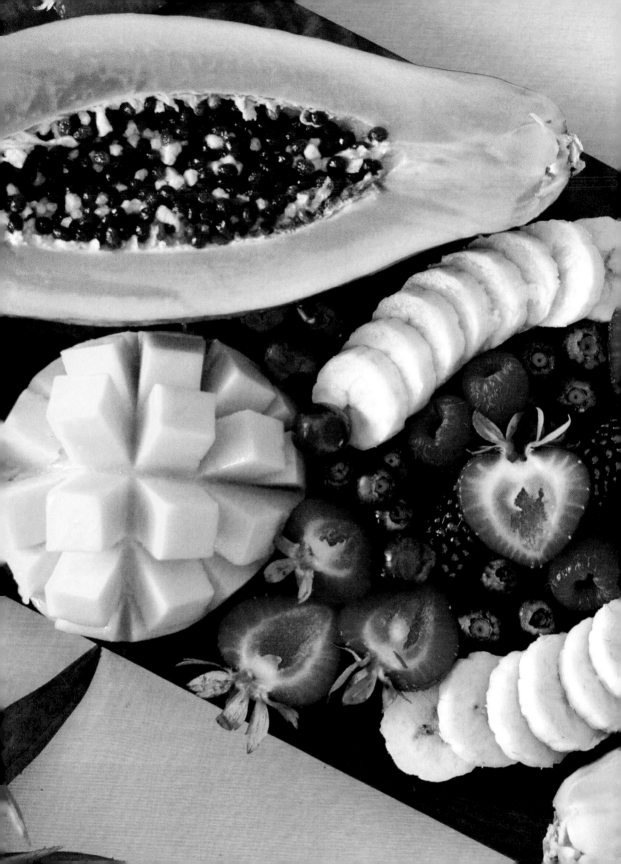

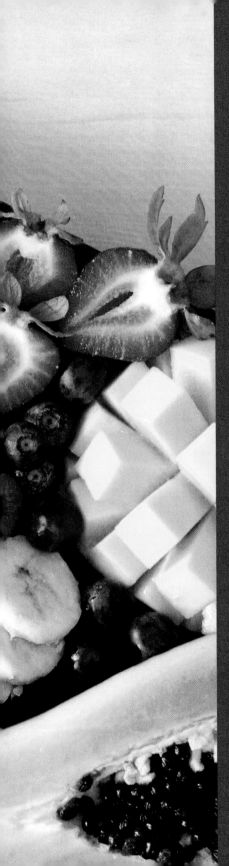

Contents

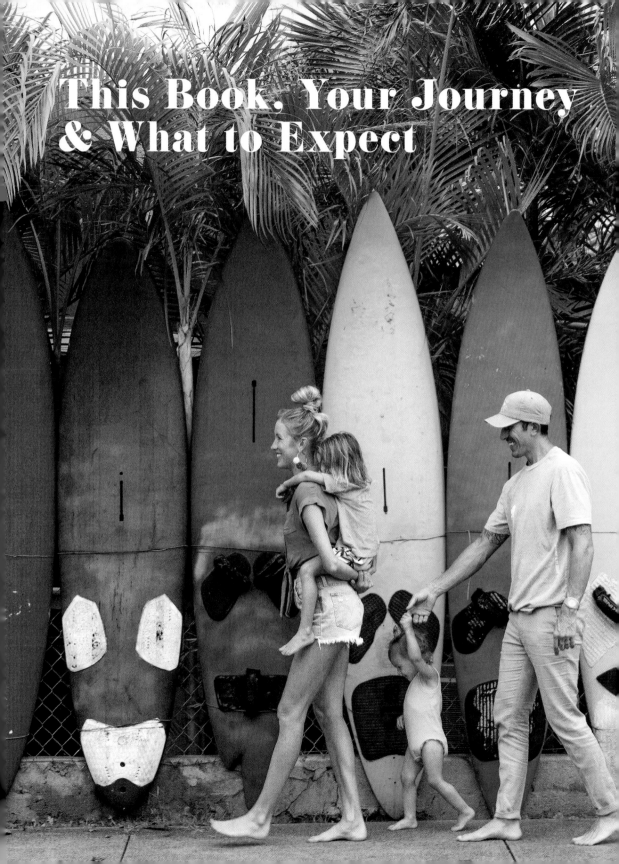

This Book, Your Journey & What to Expect

There are three basic things we all do every day, and we could all be doing them *better*: eat, move, and rest. In this book, we'll guide you through each of these basics and how to perform them with presence, intentionality, and consistency . . . a new way of living—*on purpose!*

You know how they say *hindsight is 20/20*? Well, looking back, it seems obvious now that we were on the "struggle bus" at the same time for a reason. There was a bright new path paved for us, but the road was not devoid of speed bumps. In fact, without the struggle, we would still most likely be on our old path, which was leading to destruction. We had a decision to make. Both paths were going to be bumpy, but the destinations were going to be vastly different.

I feel like we all face these fork-in-the-road moments throughout our lives. The key is to never turn back, and to know that whichever path we choose, there will always be opportunities to reroute. Don't let decision fatigue keep you stopped at the crossroads! I often say that God's plan is more like a modern-day GPS and less like an old-fashioned road map. If we make a wrong turn, He will simply reroute us. So there we went, together down a road less traveled into the unknown, with hopes for a brighter future!

While the path described in this book might be new for you, we want you to consider *The Happy Healthy Plant-Based Cookbook* your one-stop shop to better health and happiness. Focus less on pace and more on direction—*Forward!* If you approach this book with a willingness to learn, a commitment to put forth a solid effort, and an intention to lead with an open mind, you will encounter as few roadblocks as possible and immediately begin to see the results and feel the benefits this lifestyle has to offer.

Maybe you're struggling with excess weight, an illness, or a health scare. Maybe you're healthier than you've ever been and want to take things to the next level. Maybe you're curious about a plant-based lifestyle. Maybe you just want to eat cleaner. Or maybe you have young kids, too, and simply need recipes they will like. No matter why you've picked up this book, we want you to ask yourself, *Am I eating, moving, and resting my best?*

We know how confusing the health and wellness space can be. Diet wars rage on and doctors debate until they're blue in the face, but with our help, you'll be able to navigate through the confusion and simply *get back to the basics.*

The best place to start is to simply act. Dive in. Try something new and take baby steps. Bring your body and let your mind follow. You'll find the Eat Move Rest lifestyle and philosophy in the pages to follow, as well as tips, tricks, tools, and recipes to take you as far as you're willing to go.

Get ready to learn how to upgrade the foods you eat, optimize the way you move, and improve the quality of your rest.

Back to the Basics

Eat, move, rest. These simple daily tasks are essential to life as soon as we enter this big, beautiful world. Sad to say, outside influences have an immense impact on us and we often pick up bad habits before we are old enough to know better. The good news is it's never too late to course correct. Change is always possible.

The hard part is knowing which way to turn when we decide to make a change. We're sold a shiny new object on an almost daily basis—the "magic bullet" that will improve our lives forever—and if we're not careful, we can easily find ourselves weighed down beneath a pile of diet dos and don'ts, pills, potions, and obscure products that can leave us more lost than when we started.

Add to this that we're already bogged down, operating on autopilot with crammed schedules, mindless routines, and habits that don't serve us.

Here's our secret for making change happen: Do *less!*

Sometimes, like our devices, we've got to swipe our desktops clean and start fresh. We do this by getting back to the basics of how we eat, move, and rest. Once we have those basics down, we can build ourselves up to the better, upgraded, 2.0 versions of ourselves. The first step is to master what you simply can't function without:

1. **EAT more plants.**
2. **MOVE daily.**
3. **REST intentionally.**

That's it. Let's see if we can focus on *just* the basics until we have them down. The cleaner you eat, the more energy you have to move. The more you move, the better rest you'll get at night. When you wake up the next day, you'll crave the foods that gave you the energy the day before, and the cycle continues.

We call this the **Eat Move Rest Locomotive**. Like moving a train, getting started is the hardest part, but once you gain a bit of **momentum**, you become *unstoppable!* Soon, you'll reach a place where you no longer have to *think* about what to eat, how to move, and if you should slow down and rest. With a little bit of consistency, these healthy (and basic) practices become habit, and the healthy choice becomes the *easy* choice.

When you round that bend, you can more easily become the best version of yourself and show up as your best self for others. As the saying goes, "you can't pour from an empty cup." If you are continually filling your cup by the way you eat, move, and rest then you can continually do what matters most—pour out to and for those around you.

We are so grateful to have helped thousands of people around the world through our free videos on YouTube, our personal online coaching and membership group, and our in-person retreats in Costa Rica. From that small seed, Eat Move Rest has grown into nearly 200 retreat guests, more than 165,000 YouTube subscribers, millions of hours watched, multiple e-books launched, a recipe and meal-planner app, an online membership, and now this book. We love hearing how our recipes, workouts, and lifestyle habits have changed lives, and we want the same for you.

Our Stories

Present day. It's a Saturday morning. I'm woken up by the sound of the rubber feet of the barstool as it bounces against the hard tile floor. Max does his best to push and pull it across the kitchen so he can climb up and help Dad with his Saturday-morning ritual. Below the subtle hum of the juicer, I can hear Max's little voice asking, "Is this dino kale, Dad?"

The bamboo floors creak and crack under my feet as I tiptoe down the hall with baby Liv. I like to try to sneak up on the boys and watch them work together in the kitchen.

They are busy rinsing, chopping, and snapping hard stems of kale, celery, and cucumbers from the garden. It wouldn't be Saturday without a fresh-pressed green juice!

After taking a quick video of the cuteness from behind (both boys still in boxers), Liv and I join the ranks.

I'm on smoothie duty, and today I'm making a pretty pink smoothie bowl. Superfoods and seeds line the countertop, and rinsed, ripe berries are sprinkled across a tea towel. A very hungry Mr. Max bounces across the room, now sipping green juice from a bendy straw, on his way to wrestle with his furry brother and Bernese mountain dog, Beau.

Dusty and I cheers our glasses of greens and get back to work—waffles are next! We've perfected our recipe now, after more than a few failed attempts. Overall, though, I must admit learning to "veganize" any (and every) recipe has been surprisingly easy and delicious.

Who would have thought all that refined flour, sugar, and eggs could so easily be replaced by whole plant foods? Rolled oats, chia seeds, and plant milk topped with some organic Canadian-tree-tapped maple syrup . . . *Yum!*

Beyond the eye-catching colors and mouthwatering flavors, these foods also prevent, and in many cases, reverse some of the most common diseases that plague Western society. Not just a diet, my friends, this is truly a lifestyle—and one of **abundance**. Let the weekend begin!

My family lives at the crossroads between food that tastes amazing *and* makes us feel amazing . . . and the bonus is that it's *not* at all as difficult as some make it sound. In fact, with a dash of planning and pinch of preparation, it's pretty easy!

Between the two of us, Dusty and I have experienced the following health benefits by adopting a plant-based diet: more energy, increased metabolism, stellar digestion, optimal weight, better sleep, clearer skin, less brain fog, better blood work, balanced hormones, and improved mood; the list really does go on. . . . And these health benefits are important because while the breakfast-time scene I just set for you may seem idyllic—and it sure is!—there is no light without darkness.

Dusty and I found plant-based eating after some truly frightening early adulthood health scares. It took a lot of open-mindedness coupled with a hunger to learn to set us on a new path. The education we received about how to properly fuel and move our bodies, and how to rest our minds, coupled with our commitment to implementing what we learned, resulted in unimaginable growth. If we can do it, you absolutely can, too. We don't take our Saturday morning green juice ritual, or anything we're able to do daily, for granted. We feel lucky to be not just alive but *thriving*. It's our pleasure but also our *duty* to bring as many people with us as possible.

Erin's Health and Healing Journey

Let's take it back to my childhood. While my brother and I enjoyed our fair share of Happy Meals, mac 'n' cheese, and sugary beverages, my mom always made sure to balance out the "less healthy" things with fresh-fruit smoothies, juices, and plenty of home-cooked meals. My parents also made sure we stayed active, requiring us to play sports and teaching us about the importance of rest and recovery. They also held us to high academic standards. I was a straight-A, honor roll student who finished high school at the top of my class. I played varsity tennis, ran cross country, and was used to being fit. Little did I know that shortly after showing up at college much of that would change.

To put it plainly, about halfway through freshman year, I derailed. My grades weren't what they had been in high school. I was no longer staying active. And without mom around to cook I was eating worse than ever. I never had an interest in learning how to cook, so I was living on a steady diet of ramen noodles and beef jerky in my dorm room and pizza with soft serve from the cafeteria. Ever heard of the "freshman fifteen"?

My academic career took a back seat to my newfound social life, and I quickly learned I could disguise my lifetime shyness with alcohol. I began staying out late, drinking, eating fast food, and sleeping in. It didn't take long for my mental, emotional, and physical health to start slipping away, and I began to experience feelings of anxiety and depression for the first time.

Self-esteem and love is what I needed. Alcohol delivered false confidence and friends, and indulgent food felt like love. It all worked ... until it didn't. The truth is, self-esteem comes from doing "esteemable acts," as my favorite podcast host, Rich Roll, says. I was doing nothing of the sort.

I remember going for long drives in my car on Sunday mornings after three days of going out and feeling completely empty inside, tears of frustration and fear streaming down my face. My grades were suffering, my emotional health was worse than ever, and to add to the shame, I didn't even recognize myself when I looked in the mirror anymore.

I decided to start working out and eating less "junk." Monday through

Wednesday, I would exercise hard, doing hours of cardio, followed by a brief weigh-in. Then, Thursday would roll around, someone would text or knock on my door, and the party would start and often go on through the weekend.

On top of going out, I was still eating the Standard American Diet (SAD). Between drive-throughs, pizza delivery, and the dorm cafeteria, I was consuming so many unhealthy calories, I sometimes can't believe I hadn't gained more weight. I remember hearing someone in the gym say, "True health begins with what's on your fork." It made sense. I began to realize the harder I worked out, *I couldn't out-train my bad diet!*

I hate to admit that I continued this roller coaster for a couple of years. I told myself that this was normal college-kid behavior and that I was just "keeping the balance." Ha! This "balance" ended up leading me to a very dark and scary place both physically and mentally and I now know that balance, like moderation, is a very subjective term.

I began to experience a handful of symptoms including brain fog, lethargy, numbness and tingling in my extremities, and just plain exhaustion. I found myself waking up in the middle of the night breathless, and as hard as I tried, I wasn't able to get a deep enough breath, which started causing panic attacks.

My hormones were out of whack, too, so I was placed on hormonal birth control to fix my irregular menstrual cycle. While on the medication, I experienced frequent mood swings, acne, and yeast infections that often required several rounds of antibiotics. I was sad and frustrated and just wanted to feel good. In hindsight, I don't know why I was expecting to feel good when I certainly wasn't doing any good for myself.

My digestion was another issue. I was anything but regular and experienced constant bloating and gut pain. It got to a point where I was so obsessed with fiber that I was eating a steady diet of processed "fiber"-filled cereals, bars, and yogurts on the daily. I only ate packaged foods because the nutrition label could tell me exactly how many grams of fiber and calories I was consuming.

Lean Cuisine and Subway cold cuts became my new normal as I began to obsess over calories and weight loss, and while I wasn't doing great, my intentions were in the right place. I had at least recognized that my bad habits needed to change. So besides going to the gym, I started going out less and began paying more attention to the foods I was eating.

This is about the same time I reconnected with Dusty, whom I had known since high school. Not surprisingly, we bumped into each other at a bar, after finals. We exchanged details, and before we knew it, we were doing everything together. Dusty liked to cook and work out so we did both together. We started biking, going to the gym, and cooking for ourselves.

When Dusty came into the picture, he convinced me that protein was paramount. We'd start the day with scrambled eggs and hash browns. Lunch was cold-cut sub sandwiches, and dinner was some type of grilled meat or fish. No more fast food and only a little bit of pizza allowed.

After a few months of this, I had gotten back down to a healthy weight, but I still wasn't feeling great. My breathing issues, brain fog, and other symptoms persisted, and I began practicing yoga and seeing a therapist on and off to manage my crippling anxiety.

In an effort to make things better, I started doing research. "Dr." Google became my best friend *and* my worst enemy. Every symptom I searched came back with a frightening diagnosis.

I distinctly remember reading about multiple sclerosis. My symptoms matched perfectly. My heart began to race, and I felt a pit in my stomach. I had to know for sure. . . .

Coming from a family of physicians, it was easy for me to pop into my dad's office for blood work, so I did just that. From there, I met with a long list of specialists that ran an even longer list of tests from CT scans and MRIs to nerve conduction studies and extensive blood panels. No doctor could give me a diagnosis, which would seem like a relief, but I was still very much in a state of dis-ease. I hate to admit it but I actually *wanted* some kind of diagnosis, a label for a condition that could be treated to make all my problems go away.

I credit my mom for saving me. She presented Dusty and me with an opportunity to go to a series of conferences across the country to become trained and certified health and lifestyle coaches. I had recently graduated from the University of Nebraska with a degree in biology, but I had decided medical school wasn't for me. I still knew that I wanted to be able to help people heal. This became the perfect opportunity for me to (eventually) do that, but more important, it helped give me the knowledge and tools to first heal myself.

Dusty—who had just received his degree in communication and planned to

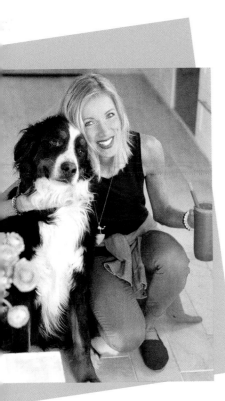

go into some type of therapy work—agreed it would be a good opportunity to learn. If nothing else, we knew it would be fun to get to travel and learn more about holistic health and wellness, so we went for it.

While completing our certifications, I found myself becoming increasingly passionate about healthy food and fitness. I recognized that the majority of attendees and speakers at the conferences were physicians and health professionals who were fed up with the traditional (diagnose and prescribe) medical system—calling it "sick-care" instead of health care. We learned a lot and met some amazing people who pushed us toward our goals for a healthier and happier future.

One afternoon, my uncle, a cardiologist, invited us to hear a physician speak at a local hospital. That person ended up being Dr. Caldwell B. Esselstyn, who was sharing his findings and success preventing and reversing heart disease in his patients by prescribing a whole food, plant-based diet to them. We had heard about this before in our conferences: a *plant-based diet*. He showed echocardiograms of patients whom he had reversed heart disease in with this way of eating, and after Dr. Esselstyn's talk, Dusty and I were so convinced that we decided to go vegetarian (not yet vegan) for the forty days of Lent.

At the end of the forty days, we were just glad to be *alive!* Dusty always jokes that the very next day, he went through the drive-through and ordered a big juicy burger—and that was not far from the truth! That being said, we began to realize how little we really relied on meat and how much better we felt without it. We decided to go back to being vegetarian as we continued to seek better health and understanding about nutrition.

It's funny now, looking back on my childhood, I never liked animal products. I would complain to my mom that the steak was too hard to cut and chew, and the milk tasted bad. And the fish filets Dusty had been grilling were never my favorite, so here I was, *finally* getting permission to cut these things out.

Without meat, though, we became *extra* obsessed with making sure we were getting enough protein. Everyone seemed to be asking us that question vegans and vegetarians get so often, "But where do you get your protein?" Our answer at the time was eggs, more eggs, and whey-protein shakes.

To track our progress toward better health, we decided to start getting regular blood work done at my parents' clinic. I remember the day when, to my surprise, the nurses gave me the news that my cholesterol was unfortunately going up. I was told that because heart disease ran in both sides of my family, it would be best for me to go on a statin drug. When I asked for how long, the response I got did not sit well. *Forever?! But I'm only in my early twenties!* That was not going to work for me, so I went back to the drawing board. Bring on the supplements, shakes, and potions. Cod-liver oil anyone? We choked it down daily, in addition to many other obscure tinctures.

While I was figuring out what I should do to get my cholesterol down, Dusty and I were still having our fun. We were young and in love so we decided to take a weekend trip to San Diego, and on that flight, I experienced a scare that shook me to my core—my rock bottom.

About an hour from landing I had a massive panic attack. My leg had gone numb from the knee down and all I could think of was multiple sclerosis or a blood clot on its way to my heart. I couldn't calm myself down and desperately asked a flight attendant if there was anything she could give me or do, which resulted in the airplane landing 30 minutes ahead of schedule. The plane raced down the jetway and was met by an ambulance, which rushed me to the emergency room. After a couple hours of tests, everything came back . . . normal. The physician evaluating me did however say some of my vitamin levels were shockingly high and mentioned I may be oversupplementing.

I was so scared but also embarrassed. The rest of the trip I struggled on and off with anxiety. When we got home. I decided it was time to get serious . . . and to get back to the basics. I tossed out my pills, potions, supplements, and even my birth control! It was time for a clean slate.

I went back to Dr. Google, but this time I was searching for *solutions* rather than symptoms.

This time, the film *Forks Over Knives* came across my radar, as well as a book titled *The China Study* (two great places to begin your plant-based journey). After devouring countless documentaries, podcasts, and blogs, I was convinced that in order to lower my cholesterol, I needed to quit consuming excess dietary cholesterol (i.e., all animal products). The simple truth is all animal products contain cholesterol and all plants do not. What plants *do* contain is fiber—and animal products do not! I decided to do what Dr. Esselstyn had suggested that day in the hospital and adopt a 100 percent whole food, plant-based diet.

After just a few weeks of eliminating eggs and eating the rainbow, my cholesterol went down to what Dr. Michael Greger (founder of NutritionFacts.org and *New York Times* bestselling author of *How Not to Die*), would call the "heart-attack-proof" range. I was *elated!* Once I realized there was an abundance of *real* fiber in every food I was now eating, my fiber obsession completely fell by the wayside.

In time, my other symptoms began to resolve, too. With perfect digestion and a cheerful disposition, I began to fully understand the gut-brain connection—food really *does* impact mood! My brain fog lifted, and I was feeling more mentally clear than ever. This boosted my confidence and helped me to feel empowered and in control of my health. I no longer experienced anxiety or panic attacks because I *knew* that my actions were in alignment with my desired outcome. Put good in, get good out.

By the time Dusty and I had become certified health and lifestyle coaches, I was feeling better than I ever had. I was at a place in my life where I was really trying hard to figure out who I was and how I fit into the world. I decided I would start sharing what had helped me get back to the basics and become the healthiest, happiest version of myself. Shortly after, Eat Move Rest, our online-community and lifestyle brand, was born!

Flash Forward: Yes, we are now parents to three little ones, and I know there can be a lot of questions and concerns around how to have a healthy plant-based pregnancy and postpartum period. More on that part of my journey on page 23.

Dusty's Health and Healing Journey

My journey began with resistance. I was a Midwest boy, brought up in a culture of football, beef, and beers. As a kid, I played backyard football games with my buddies that often ended in a bloody nose or fistfight and watched the neighborhood dads drink, yell, and grill. It was all about being tough.

As I grew, so did my appetite. While my mom's meals at home had always been healthy, once I had my driver's license, it was game on. Drive-throughs and pizza joints for lunch were followed by Friday night grill-outs with my friends. I had a buddy who worked at the neighborhood grocery store, and he would bring each of us a piece of meat. The bigger the better, and whoever ate the most proved he was the most "manly."

I often tell guys who are trying to get healthy this part of my story and admit I never thought I would eat the plant-based way. I certainly never *wanted* to eat this way, but now, I can't imagine living any other way. But, unlike Erin, at that time, I wasn't going to make any changes until I *had* to, so I took my sweet time.

Besides my own fears about not getting enough protein and losing weight or muscle, I was *more* concerned about what my buddies would think of me. I was concerned what my cattle-farming uncle and hunter grandpa would think of their "vegetarian" grandson. What I needed was *permission*. And I remember right where I was when I got it.

I was lying on our bed one evening researching plant-based diets and protein, when I found a *Forks Over Knives* article written by Rich Roll. It was called "Slaying the Protein Myth," and in the opening lines he states, "I am plant-based. I'm also an ultra-endurance athlete." He got me.

By the end of the article, I had not only gotten the "permission" I needed to pursue this new way of eating, I also felt pumped up about doing it. I was excited for the possibilities and ready for the challenge. This was a major turning point in my health and healing journey, which began about as early as it could.

When I was just a year old, my parents began to notice I was having trouble with my left leg. I was walking but only on my tiptoes on the left side. After some testing, doctors confirmed I had been born with a mild case of cerebral palsy. Cerebral palsy is associated with movement and coordination problems and in my case appeared to only affect the left side of my body, and specifically my left leg. It was about a half inch shorter than my right one and skinnier, twisted in, and pointed down.

My parents were assured that while things would typically not get better, they would not get worse as long as the right steps were taken, no pun intended. And so it began! My first shoes, a white pair of Reebok tennies, were fitted with an extra-thick outer sole on the left side to compensate for my discrepancy.

I recently stumbled upon that first pair of shoes and had to laugh at how heavy that left shoe was! I imagined my little one-year old self trying to get around with that heavy thing around my weak leg. It definitely would have been making me stronger!

For the next few years, I was busy with physical therapy and doctor visits. In an attempt to fix my irregular gait, I was outfitted with a terribly uncomfortable brace, and since I was always outgrowing the brace, I had to get new ones made all the time. I dreaded those appointments. As if the wet plaster mold wasn't uncomfortable enough, the doctor used a scary-looking saw-type tool with a two-inch spinning blade to cut the hardened mold off.

But soon, the braces and heavy outsoles were replaced with rubber insoles, which were less noticeable to the outside world, thank goodness.

As I got older, I got stronger. My physical therapy helped a lot, and by third grade I was able to say goodbye to Birdie, my therapist, and continue my therapy alone.

To this day, stretching is still a part of my routine. I get up from the floor, as instructed, with my "left leg only" and often catch myself reciting in my head "heel toe, heel toe" every time I walk in public.

This journey made me strong, resilient, and wise. I had to work a little harder and be a little bit more conscientious than my peers. I fought hard to be the fastest kid on the playground. My parents insisted I wasn't any different. They expected great things from me and never accepted excuses. As a result, I was an athlete and good student and a solid big brother.

As challenging as all this was, these experiences made me who I am and instilled in me an attitude of gratitude for simple things, like two working legs. They taught me to find solutions. Doing hard things was my "normal." These lessons have served me well in adulthood and during my wellness transformation.

By freshman year of college, my good grades and admirable behavior had gone out the window. Similar to Erin, I partied myself right out of my fraternity and into academic probation.

I never felt good. I was terribly anxious and often depressed. I lived a very dark and lonely life even though I was surrounded by people and parties. To make things worse, I was always sick. Sinus infection after sinus infection and antibiotic after antibiotic for two years, until I had surgery to have my adenoids removed.

After finally getting sick and tired of *being* sick and tired, I decided to move home for my last year (or so) of college. My parents had recently gone through a devastating divorce. My mom, who had never worked a day in her life, suddenly found herself alone raising my little brother and providing for all three of us. Moving home just felt right, so I did.

I stopped partying (as much) and started eating better. I had always enjoyed cooking, and now I had a clean and well-stocked kitchen to do it in. I had also always loved cycling from my BMX days as a kid, so biking became my form of regular fitness. I was feeling okay!

I cut out most fast food and made eggs for breakfast, turkey sandwiches for lunch, and grilled pork chops or tilapia for dinner. For dessert I would have Little Debbie Zebra Cakes and a tall glass of whole milk followed by buttered toast or a cream cheese bagel for a midnight snack.

Despite some nagging heartburn, I was feeling pretty good, healthwise. I was feeling pretty good about life, too. I was about to finish and earn my bachelor's degree with a high GPA.

Enter Erin.

We bumped into each other in a bar after finals, and while we were bonding over beers at the time, we shared with each our desires to get healthier.

We were then, and still are, optimizers, always searching for the best and most efficient way of doing things: food, fitness, and beyond. I instantly fell in love with Erin's energy and ambition to do, be, and feel better, and my commitment to staying single forever started to diminish.

Shortly after Erin's wake-up call in San Diego, I decided I also needed to address some of my own health issues.

I had been dealing with acid reflux that was getting progressively worse. The doctor's advice for "managing" reflux was to avoid spicy food, eat hard-boiled eggs, and drink whole cow's milk.

When that didn't help, I was put on a PPI or "proton pump inhibitor" to basically turn off the acid in my stomach. It seemed harmless at the time, and it worked. My acid reflux was gone, and as advertised, I could continue eating what I wanted, without the discomfort.

After a year on the drug, the reflux started creeping back in. The doctor prescribed another medication so I took it. When the reflux still wouldn't go away, I was told to add a *third medication*. I stopped to think, *If I'm already taking this many pills in my midtwenties, how many pills would I be taking by the time I was thirty or forty? Are these things even safe? And how much money is this going to cost me each month?* I quickly did the math. *For the REST OF MY LIFE!?* My head started to spin!

Like Erin, I firmly believe God had us on this path together for a reason. Both of us were in a similar place when we started down a scary new road that would soon become one of the best decisions I have *ever* made.

A Turning Point for Us Both

Erin and I made the decision to get certified as health and lifestyle coaches together, and we got to work, attending lecture after lecture taught by an impressive collection of academics, medical doctors, and scientists who were fighting for a new model of health and wellness.

We learned about the benefits of fasting, compared the vitamin levels in cooked versus raw food, and discovered that implementing simple changes, such as drinking more water, breathing more deeply, and stretching, could be game changers. Mindful eating really blew us away!

During one exercise, we were told to go and grab a piece of (vegetarian) food from the lunch spread and imagine its lifespan: where it was planted; the farmer who spent months watering it; the people who picked, packed, and shipped it to a grocery store; and even the grocery clerk who handled and sold it. We practiced gratitude for all those hands that went into bringing this food to ours now. Then we were told to eat using only our hands. No forks or utensils. We realized that this is not only a very primal but safe way of eating. You'll never burn your mouth if you touch your food with your hands first! I did feel bad for people who chose spaghetti, though!

Finally, we were told to chew each bite at least twenty times. Chewing this much would make sure the enzymes in our mouths and guts could properly digest our food. Talk about slow food! That was the longest lunch break we'd ever had but also the most profound eating experience of our lives. Ever since, our eating practice has included mindfulness and practicing gratitude.

While everything we learned during these years had an impact on us, only a couple of lecturers had encouraged a *fully* plant-based diet . . . until that day we met Dr. Esselstyn.

He was completely reversing heart disease with a simple, safe, and affordable protocol: a plant-based diet. *A what!?* I thought, and then the food came out: bean sprout quesadillas with hummus spread and sliced veggies. The vibe was academic conference meets hippie vegan festival. The truth is, we were digging it!

The information was irrefutable, and the food was *actually* delicious. On our drive home that day, we agreed to give it a shot—and so started our forty-day journey to health. We adopted a "plant-based diet" for Lent that year, and while it was challenging at first, we had never felt better! My reflux? Gone! Erin's cholesterol at her next checkup, down! There was really something to this diet.

Erin stayed committed and went full speed into this new way of eating, and I'm so glad she did. We unpacked the blender we had received as a wedding gift and started making smoothies. Our morning scrambled eggs got replaced with a "salad in a glass" as Erin calls it.

That green smoothie gave us energy, helped us poop, helped lower Erin's cholesterol, and fixed my damaged gut. At a time when I still hadn't committed to a fully plant-based diet, *this* was my lifeline. We began sharing the smoothie recipe with friends and family, encouraging anyone who wanted to make a small step toward better health to give it a try. One day, Erin decided to share her recipe on social media and got such a great response that she started sharing more, from plant-based lunch salads to hearty plant-based dinners.

As the number of likes and followers grew, we realized we could be doing more with this content. I remember sitting at our little high-top dinner table in our tiny apartment trying to come up with names for the brand.

"Back to the basics," Erin kept saying. "It can't be *just* food." We wanted to take a more holistic approach, knowing that wellness was more than what was on our plate. "What are the three things we do every day for our health?" Erin asked.

I replied, "We all have to eat, we *should* be moving our bodies, and we definitely need quality rest."

"That's it! Eat Move Rest," Erin declared, and we purchased the online domain that night!

From there, we started building our website, formulating a mission statement, and getting to work. Erin dove in headfirst designing the website and writing blog posts. Many months passed before the site was up and running, and it would be many more until anyone besides our moms was visiting the blog. Thanks moms!

Inspired by her favorite food blogger, Erin decided she would start posting the recipes on this new app that was growing in popularity—Instagram. The online community was born, and the rest is history!

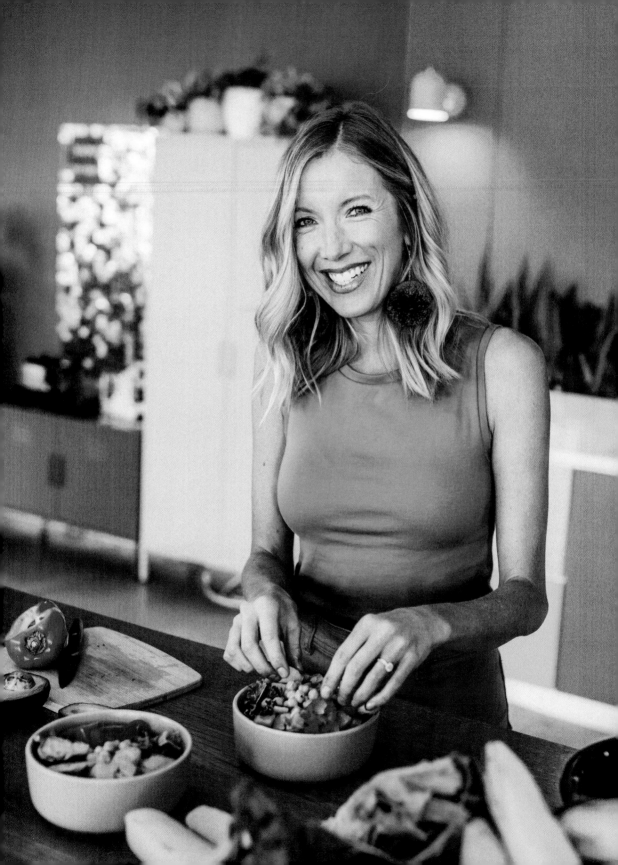

Part One

How to Eat Move Rest Your Best

We could all be happier and healthier if we ate more plants, moved our bodies daily, and got quality rest. There are many ways to approach each of these, but we're going to share the ones that we've found to be the most effective, enjoyable, and, most important, *sustainable*.

We think that when it comes to health, its best to take a holistic approach. Just as a single organ can't operate outside of the body and a car can't run without an engine, we can't operate as the best versions of ourselves if we aren't addressing our body and mind as a whole. Getting back to the basics is a whole *lifestyle*.

The destination is not as important as the journey, a continual quest to discover and empower ourselves with upgraded ways of eating, moving, and resting. As we explore, our physical health improves and we become more mentally clear and better able to do the "inner work." We peel back the onion layers to reveal deeper and more meaningful parts of our truest selves.

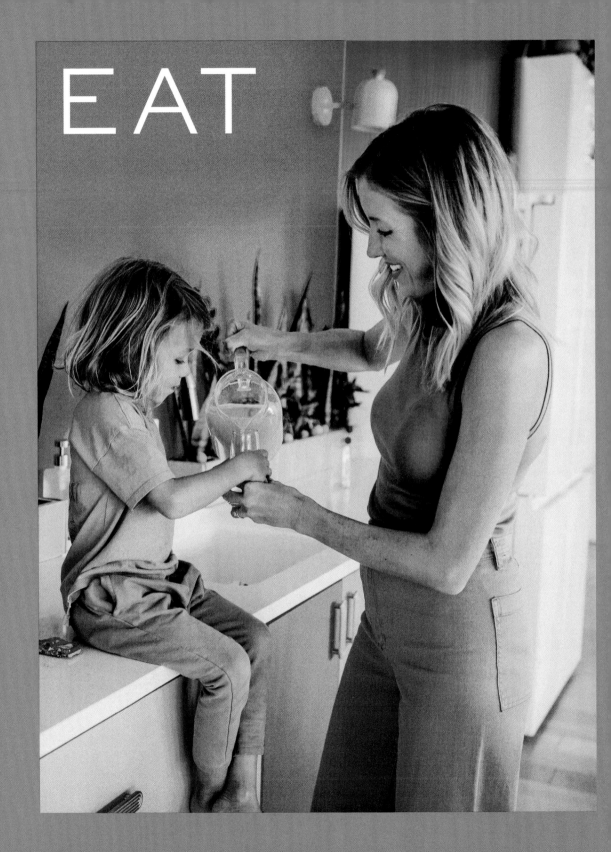

EAT

We start with "Eat" because we all must do it multiple times a day. Food is fuel, but it's also something to be enjoyed. Food is what we bond over and create rich memories around—and as such, we shouldn't have to sacrifice our health to do so. What we eat can make us or break us, and a whole food, plant-based diet is a great entry point to a healthier and, ultimately, happier life!

The Essentials

We recommend consuming plant foods as close to their natural state as possible. The essentials include the following:

- Fruits and veggies (Lots of them and in every color of the rainbow!)
- Whole grains
- Beans and legumes
- Nuts and seeds
- Herbs and spices

*Note: Check out the Plant-Based Essentials Grocery List on page 10 for an idea of just how much variety this entails!

To an outsider, a plant-based diet might seem limiting, but we have found it to be quite the opposite. We eat so much more variety now than on the SAD (Standard American Diet). For example, there are hundreds of types of beans and legumes we never even knew existed. Hunting down and trying new, exotic fruit varieties is one of our favorite things to do when we travel. If you "live to eat," this diet is for you—plant foods are generally lower in calories but higher in volume, fiber, and water, which means you get to eat in *abundance* and feel satiated rather than deprived.

Our FAQ

Where do you get your protein?

We will make this easy: we get it from plants! All plant foods contain protein, and many are "complete proteins," meaning they contain all nine essential amino acids (the ones that our bodies don't make and we must obtain from our diet). Some complete plant proteins that we commonly enjoy are quinoa, soy, chia seeds, spirulina, hemp seeds, buckwheat, and amaranth.

The body can function optimally on plant proteins. It doesn't matter to the body where your protein comes from—but what does matter are the other nutrients contained in the protein "package."[1] Many animal-based forms of protein come with dietary cholesterol and excess saturated fat that are linked to higher risks of cancer, diabetes, and weight gain.[2]

Animal protein may negatively influence long-term health, so we get our protein from plants. Plant-based protein sources do not contain undesirable components, rather they include phytonutrients, antioxidants, and fiber, which are all linked to lower risks of cancer, heart disease, and diabetes.[3] Fiber promotes good gut bacteria, smoother digestion, and improved heart health.[4]

Bonus: Plant proteins are good for the body *and* the planet. In terms of land use, freshwater consumption, and greenhouse gas emissions, plant foods use way fewer resources than animal products.[5] An added bonus: When you opt for proteins that grew in the ground—not on a feedlot—your conscience can rest easy about animal cruelty concerns.

---

[1] P. J. Skerrett and W. C. Willett, "Essentials of Healthy Eating: A Guide," *Journal of Midwifery and Women's Health* 55, no. 6 (November–December 2010): 492–501, https://doi.org/10.1016/j.jmwh.2010.06.019.

[2] "Animal Protein and Cancer Risk," Osher Center for Integrative Health, University of California San Francisco, https://osher.ucsf.edu/patient-care/integrative-medicine-resources/cancer-and-nutrition/faq/animal-protein-cancer-risk.

[3] R. T. Ahnen, S. S. Jonnalagadda, and J. L. Slavin, "Role of Plant Protein in Nutrition, Wellness, and Health," *Nutrition Reviews* 77, no. 11 (November 2019), 735–47, https://doi.org/10.1093/nutrit/nuz028.

[4] "Dietary Fiber: Essential for a Healthy Diet," Mayo Clinic, posted November 4, 2022, https://www.mayoclinic.org/healthy-lifestyle/nutrition-and-healthy-eating/in-depth/fiber/art-20043983; Julie Corliss, "How a Fiber-Rich Diet Promotes Heart Health," posted August 1, 2022, https://www.health.harvard.edu/heart-health/how-a-fiber-rich-diet-promotes-heart-health.

[5] "Animal-Based Foods Are More Resource-Intensive than Plant-Based Foods," World Resources Institute, posted April 20, 2016, https://www.wri.org/data/animal-based-foods-are-more-resource-intensive-plant-based-foods.

Will a plant-based diet increase my fiber intake?

Yes! While most people are concerned about protein intake, we should really be focused on fiber.

As Dr. Michael Greger has pointed out, studies have found that while 97 percent of Americans get enough protein—including vegans and vegetarians who average 70 percent more protein than the recommended average requirement—only 3 percent are getting enough fiber![6] But do you know who is getting plenty of fiber, found in abundance in all plant foods? People eating a completely plant-based diet and even semivegetarians! Want to increase overall gut health, digestion, elimination, skin health, and even cardiovascular health?[7] Eat more plants and get more fiber.

If I go plant-based, should I load up on plant-based food alternatives, like veggie burgers?

Countless companies are jumping on board, slapping the "vegan" label on their products as a selling point. While, yes, it is better for the animals and the planet, many of these foods are highly processed and may not be doing your body any more good than consuming animal products or fast food. A store-bought veggie burger is a nice stepping stone if you're eliminating meat, but it's best if these types of foods are used as a transition tool to get you moving toward a plant-based diet of mostly whole foods—foods that have been processed as little as possible. Think fresh fruits and veggies and whole grains. When you're ready, dabble in making your own bean and veggie burgers at home. (Try our epic Bountiful Black Bean Veggie Burgers on page 141!)

Besides limiting animal-based foods, are there any other foods I should avoid?

We recommend minimizing salt, oils, and refined sugar—also referred to as SOS foods. These three ingredients are often found in prepared and packaged foods, which is why these foods are typically higher in calories and lower in nutrition and cause us to crave *even more of them!* Foods high in salt, oils, and refined sugar

---

[6] Michael Greger, "Where Do You Get Your Fiber?," Nutrition Facts (blog), last updated September 25, 2023, https://nutritionfacts.org/blog/where-do-you-get-your-fiber.

[7] Allison Dilzer, Julie Jones, and Marie E. Latulippe, "The Family of Dietary Fibers: Dietary Variety for Maximum Health Benefit," *Nutrition Today* 48, no. 3 (May/June 2013): 108–18, https:doi.org/10.1097/NT.0b013e3182941d82.

can cause inflammation, spikes in blood sugar, clogged arteries, high blood pressure, and eventually, many diseases that are plaguing our country.[8]

The cool thing about eating more plants is that your taste buds will adjust. Our sugar cravings are satisfied with fruit, and foods like celery give our dinners and salads the right amount of saltiness. But we are not purists, and we do occasionally cook with these ingredients.

But wait . . . are you vegan?
Or plant-based? What's the difference?

We consider ourselves to be both! If you were unaware there was a difference, the short and simple answer is that veganism encompasses more than just omitting animal products from your diet. At its core, it's about nonharm and compassion for all living beings, essentially animal welfare and equality. Being "plant-based" is generally diet-specific. You could be plant-based and still wear leather, but a vegan would do their best to avoid animal products outside of the food world, such as leather, silk, and fur. That being said, a "vegan" diet, isn't always a healthy one. You could technically consume only canned peaches and French fries and call yourself vegan. We wouldn't recommend that!

So, is being "whole food, plant-based," or "vegan" better?

Here's the coolest part: being *all three* is best. Most people enter into this lifestyle for ethical reasons or health purposes. Being whole food, plant-based, and vegan is better for your health, better for the animals, *and* better for the planet. It's a win-win-win!

Keep in mind that despite what some people might try to tell you, you don't have to be 100 percent plant-based or vegan. There is a sliding scale, and we say you've got to find where you feel best on that scale. Anywhere you can get closer to eating more plants and fewer animals, the better!

The main thing is acknowledging your own process and the process of others. These labels, like many, can often be more exclusionary than inclusive, so we try to steer clear and encourage and acknowledge individuals to come as they are.

---

[8] "5 Types of Foods That Cause Inflammation," Cleveland Clinic, posted April 29, 2024, https://health.clevelandclinic.org/5-foods-that-can-cause-inflammation.

Plant-Based Food Pyramid and Plate

The biggest myth that we had to shake from our psyche is that protein is paramount. Once our eyes were opened to the fact that we're getting way more protein than we need, we chose to focus on our body's preferred fuel source, glycogen.

Where do we get glycogen? From the one place we've all been conditioned to fear and avoid like the plague—yes, the *carb*! Carbohydrates are broken down into glucose (or blood sugar) and our bodies (and brains) *run* on glucose! Not all carbs are created equal, though. There is a big difference between refined carbohydrates—found in foods such as white bread, doughnuts, baked goods, and pasta—and unrefined carbohydrates. Many of these foods containing refined carbohydrates have been stripped of their fiber and likely contain a not-so-healthy dose of white table sugar. We eat primarily unrefined carbohydrates from whole food sources, such as potatoes, sweet potatoes, fresh fruit, vegetables, and whole grains. These are filled with beneficial fiber, vitamins, and minerals.

Plant foods, perfectly designed and packaged by nature, provide the best amounts of the three macronutrients we need: protein, carbohydrates, and fat. The majority of plant foods are overwhelmingly rich in carbohydrates and lower in protein and fat. The beauty is, rather than worrying too much about your macronutrient ratio and hitting certain percentages, you can eat freely and in abundance, knowing that nature designed us to eat this way.

We suggest you use the Plant-Based Pyramid (page 8) to help you build your plate for each meal, filling up on the fruits and vegetables at the base of the pyramid. We place an emphasis on the most colorful and freshest foods and encourage you to eat as many raw and minimally processed fruits and vegetables as possible, followed by whole grains, then legumes, beans, and superfoods, such as wheatgrass, nutritional yeast, and goji berries.

At the very top of the pyramid, we place healthy fats, primarily avocados, nuts, and seeds.

While oils, such as olive oil, do have some benefits, we choose not to consume them and opt for whole food options instead. Eat the avocado, not the avocado oil! Oil is the most calorically dense food on the planet, and it's stripped of fiber, water, vitamins, and minerals. We feel that the drawbacks outweigh the potential benefits, especially when we have access to an abundance of healthy omega-3-rich, whole plant foods!

plant-based
pyramid

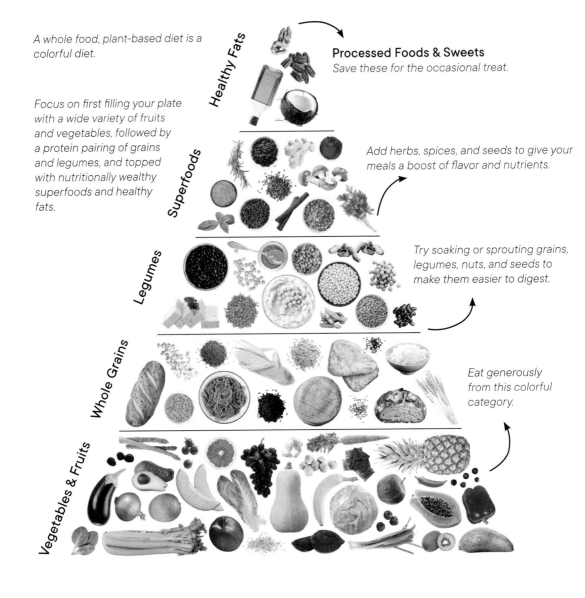

A whole food, plant-based diet is a colorful diet.

Focus on first filling your plate with a wide variety of fruits and vegetables, followed by a protein pairing of grains and legumes, and topped with nutritionally wealthy superfoods and healthy fats.

Healthy Fats

Processed Foods & Sweets
Save these for the occasional treat.

Superfoods

Add herbs, spices, and seeds to give your meals a boost of flavor and nutrients.

Legumes

Try soaking or sprouting grains, legumes, nuts, and seeds to make them easier to digest.

Whole Grains

Eat generously from this colorful category.

Vegetables & Fruits

Plant-Based Essentials Grocery List

The key to shopping healthfully is to put your blinders on and shop the perimeter. Most unhealthy options are sandwiched in the middle aisles of the store. Start at the produce section for fruits and veggies, hit up the bulk bins nearby to stock up on whole grains, beans, legumes, nuts, and seeds, and then loop back around to the frozen foods section for more fruits (great for smoothies!) and vegetables, and you should have most of what you need!

If you're new to a whole food, plant-based diet, we recommend *adding before you subtract*. Rather than wiping your fridge clean of all animal foods and packaged products, begin by adding some new produce items to your shopping cart the next time you go to the store.

Incorporate more of the whole foods you already love, enjoy, and know how to prepare. Add some extra berries and bananas to your cart so you can top your morning oatmeal with them or experiment with some of our delicious smoothie recipes.

Stock your pantry with a new type of whole grain. If you're used to rice, try quinoa! A simple swap can make a world of difference to a familiar dish.

Learn to cook with spices and herbs. Many of our soups and stews—especially the Indian- and Thai-inspired ones—will give you an opportunity to start incorporating more herbs and spices and to fall in love with a whole new level of flavor. Additionally, many spices and herbs, such as turmeric and ginger, have been found to have anti-inflammatory and other health benefits.

We stock up on jarred (avoid canned, if possible, to limit your exposure to BPA and other potentially toxic can linings) tomatoes and pastes for Italian nights; tamari and coconut aminos for stir-fry; nutritional yeast for cheesy flavor; and hummus, nut, and seed butters to create delicious sauces and salad dressings.

Here are some of our insider tips:

- **Opt for plant-based milks in the refrigerated section.** We don't think plant-based milks are essential, but the ones in the refrigerated section tend to contain less additives and preservatives. We like oat milk best for its taste and soy milk best for its nutritional profile (lots of protein and healthy fat). Select a fortified version for an added boost of vitamins and

These are the staple foods we stock up on each week at the grocery store:

FRESH FRUIT	FRESH VEGETABLES		HERBS	FROZEN FOODS	GRAINS/ BEANS
Apples	Arugula	Mushrooms	Basil	Açaí	Amaranth
Bananas	Avocado	Potatoes	Cilantro	Berries	Black beans
Berries	Beets	Radishes	Mint	Edamame	Brown rice
Lemon	Bell peppers	Red cabbage	Parsley	Green peas	Chickpeas
Lime	Carrots	Red onion		Mango	Ezekiel bread
Mandarins	Cauliflower	Romaine		Pitaya	GF pasta
Mango	Celery	Spinach		Sweet corn	Green lentils
Melon	Cherry tomatoes	Squash			Millet
Nectarines	Collards	Sweet potatoes			Quinoa
Oranges	Cucumber	Tomatoes			Red lentils
Papaya	Dino kale	Turmeric root			Rolled oats
Peaches	Garlic	Yellow onions			Steel-cut oats
Pineapple	Gingerroot	Zucchini			Tortillas
	Green onions				
	Green-leaf lettuce				

SPICES	CONDIMENTS	NUTS & SEEDS	MISC.	SUPERFOODS
Black peppercorn	Coconut aminos	Almonds	Canned tomatoes	Açaí
Chili powder	Curry paste	Cashews	Coconut milk	Barley powder
Cinnamon	Hot sauce	Chia	Coconut sugar	Cacao
Cumin	Hummus	Flax	Dates	Maca
Curry powder	Sauerkraut	Hemp	Herbal teas	Spirulina
Dulse flakes	Tamari	Nut/seed butter*	Maple syrup	
Garlic powder		Pumpkin seeds	Nondairy milk	
Ground turmeric		Sunflower seeds	Nondairy yogurt	
Italian herbs		Walnuts	Protein powder	
Nutritional yeast			Tempeh	
Onion powder			Tofu	
Sea salt			Tomato paste	
			Tomato puree	
			Vegetable broth	

* (e.g. almond butter, cashew butter, peanut butter, tahini)

minerals such as B^{12}, D, and calcium. If you want to make your own, check out our Creamy Vanilla Plant Milk (page 75).

- **Choose wraps, breads, bagels, and tortillas from the frozen foods section.** Like refrigerated milks, breads that are kept frozen typically don't contain many preservatives. If they were sitting on the shelf next to the standard white bread, they'd be all mold! We keep our organic sprouted Ezekiel bread refrigerated or frozen and just use the defrost setting on our toaster when preparing.
- **Snack smart.** If you're feeling the need for a packaged snack and/or have kiddos to please, look for bars with zero added sugar (think, dates and nuts) and crackers made without oil that contain healthy omega-3-rich seeds.

The Eat Move Rest Tool Chest

To gain access to the Eat Move Rest Tool Chest, join the Eat Move Rest Club at membership.eatmoverest.com. Inside, you'll find e-books and guides as well as a bustling community and our meal planner and recipe app!

Head over to EatMoveRest.com to find our favorite kitchen and personal care products plus discounts codes.

A Note on Processed Foods: Are They All Bad?

No! *Phew!* It's important to keep in mind that not all processed foods are created equally. For example, pasta is "processed," but the process itself is far less involved than that of something like a doughnut, box of cookies, or bag of chips. Many labels will try to lure you in with the "vegan" label, but that doesn't necessarily automatically make it a "health food."

When reading a food label, less is more. A good quality pasta will contain a couple of ingredients and sometimes just one (i.e. red lentil and brown rice or just chickpeas). These foods have been minimally processed and have not been stripped of fiber and other beneficial nutrients.

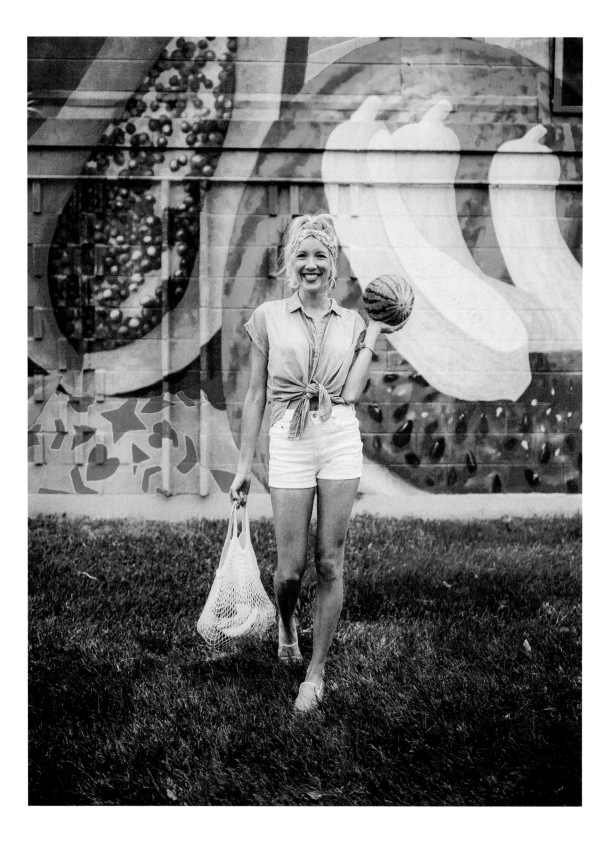

Another great example of a minimally processed whole food is oats. There is a sliding scale with the least processed (fully intact) being whole oat groats, then steel-cut oats, then rolled oats, and finally, oat flour. These foods are all still part of a healthy whole food, plant-based diet that we consume and will be used regularly in this book.

Generally speaking, if you can't read it, don't eat it. Look out for ingredients that sound like "Franken-foods," such as partially hydrogenated corn or soybean oil (trans fats) and dextrose and sucrose (code for sugar). They've typically been engineered in a lab and are strategically designed to keep you craving more.

Remember to minimize or avoid the SOS foods:

- **Salt**. If the milligrams of salt exceed the calories per serving, rethink your purchase.
- **Oil**. Particularly trans fats, excess saturated fat, and soybean oil, which is often genetically modified.
- **Sugar**. Especially high-fructose corn syrup and artificial sweeteners such as aspartame.

Kitchen Appliances and Tools List

These are the kitchen essentials we use and love:

- **Chef's knife.** This is the #1 tool to help you to succeed on a plant-based lifestyle. It doesn't have to break the bank, just make sure it's sharp!
- **Cutting board.** Look for a wooden one that's large and sturdy.
- **High-speed blender.** If you're cooking for one, a single-serving-size blender like the Nutribullet will work best. But if you're feeding a crowd, we highly recommend a Vitamix blender. We started out thinking that our budget wouldn't allow for one and burned up several less expensive blenders before we decided it was time to upgrade. The investment was well worth it because it's a versatile machine that will last you a lifetime

and it will give you a superior smoothie and "nice cream" blend, which adds to the enjoyment of your meals.

- **Pressure cooker (like an Instant Pot).** When we made the shift from buying canned beans to cooking dried beans, we couldn't have stuck with it without our pressure cooker. It also works great for steaming and slow-cooking stews, and it actually preserves more nutrients than stovetop cooking. (See how we pressure-cook our beans on page 118.)

Other favorites include:

- **Water purifier.** Opt for a filter that at least gets rid of chlorine and fluoride, but reverse osmosis filtration is optimal.
- **Food processor.** Great for making salsas, gazpachos, hummus, and finely shredded veggies.
- **Dutch oven.** Perfect for large soups, stews, curries, and even oatmeal.
- **Air fryer.** An efficient way to make oil-free potato wedges, sweet fries, and cubed tofu.

What about a juicer?

We do own a juicer, but we only use it one to two times per week. We tend to think of juicing as something we do to heal and save it for medicinal purposes. When we're feeling under the weather or weighed down, a good green juice does the trick. If you do invest in a juicer, we recommend a slow cold-press, centrifugal juicer. It extracts the maximum amount of juice with the least oxidation and damage to your produce.

Simple Swaps and Easy Upgrades

If you're feeling stuck as you go to recreate one of your favorite meals, try these plant-powered replacements!

INSTEAD OF	TRY
OIL	• Sautéing in a splash of water or vegetable broth • Baking with nut butter, applesauce, or mashed bananas • Whole food fats like avocado, nuts, and seeds to make a dish richer and creamier
REFINED SUGARS	• Pitted Medjool dates to sweeten oats, waffles, baked goods, and smoothies • Maple syrup • Coconut sugar
GLUTEN / WHEAT	• Chickpea, lentil, or brown rice pasta • Oat flour for baking • If you don't have celiac disease, simply try upgrading to an organic sprouted whole wheat or sourdough bread for easier digestion (We like Ezekiel bread.)
SOY	• Homemade Red Lentil Tofu (page 117) • Pea, hemp, or rice milk
TABLE SALT	• Sea salt or celery salt
EGGS	• Tofu to make scramble • Chia seeds or flaxseeds for baking • Applesauce as a fat-free option for baking
DAIRY	• Soy, pea, hemp, or oat milk or our Creamy Vanilla Plant Milk (page 75) • Fortified plant milks are an option, just look for milks without added sugar, fillers, and gums • Creamy Cashew Cheeze (page 219) • Nutritional yeast gives a cheesy and nutty flavor for sauces or topping salads and soups
MEAT	• Lentils for high protein and iron and a "meaty" texture; try Tasty Lentil Quinoa Tacos (page 170) and Spaghetti and Meat(less) Balls (page 174) • Beans and chickpeas for protein and iron; try our Bountiful Black Bean Veggie Burgers (page 141) and Chickpea Falafel Patties (page 142) • Tofu for protein and iron; try the ground tofu (sofritas) in our Better-for-You Burrito Balance Bowl (page 116)

Essential Nutrients and Potential Supplements

NUTRIENT	SUPPORTS	PLANT-BASED SOURCES
PROTEIN	cell repair and formation, muscle and bone building and repair, hormone and enzyme production	hemp, tofu, tempeh, seaweed, spirulina, lentils, beans, chickpeas, quinoa, oats, pumpkin seeds, chia seeds, buckwheat, peas, nutritional yeast, clean protein powder
IRON	red blood cell formation, oxygen transport, immune function, growth and development, enzyme formation, DNA synthesis, hormone formation **Pairing vitamin C–rich foods with iron-rich foods can aid in proper iron absorption.**	seaweed, sesame seeds, hemp seeds, chia seeds, cashews, flaxseeds, sunflower seeds, oats, spinach, lentils, amaranth, chickpeas, kidney beans, soybeans, pumpkin seeds
CALCIUM	strong bones, heart health, muscle and nerve function **Calcium absorption can be optimized by pairing with vitamin D–rich foods.**	soybeans, sesame seeds, chia seeds, flaxseeds, almonds, kale, collards, arugula, spinach, beans, peas, lentils, almonds
ZINC	immune system, DNA synthesis, wound healing, growth and development, carbohydrate metabolism	cashews, chia seeds, Brazil nuts, almonds, buckwheat, chickpeas, black beans, pumpkin seeds, legumes
OMEGA-3	heart health, brain health, eye health, skin health, joint health	**best to supplement DHA/EPA;** flaxseeds, chia seeds, hemp seeds, walnuts, spirulina, edamame, tofu
IODINE	thyroid health, metabolism, growth of bones and nerves	sea veggies (dulse, wakame), potatoes (w/ skin), iodized salt
SELENIUM	reproductive health, thyroid health, DNA synthesis, healing from infection and oxidative stress	Brazil nuts, lentils, cashews, spinach, sunflower seeds, tofu, whole wheat bread
VITAMIN B^{12}	proper nervous system function, red blood cell formation, DNA synthesis, energy, sleep, anemia prevention, heart health	**best to supplement;** fortified foods, bacteria found in soil
VITAMIN D^3	bone health, immune function, calcium absorption, healing from infection, heart health, mood regulation, reduced inflammation, cancer prevention	**best to supplement;** fortified foods, sunshine
VITAMIN K	bone health, blood clotting, memory, heart health **Vitamin K should be taken with Vitamin D in order to properly metabolize calcium for building bone.**	asparagus, broccoli, Brussels sprouts, kale and other dark leafy greens, sauerkraut, tempeh, soybeans, blueberries, grapes
VITAMIN A	energy production, nerve function, immune system function, red blood cell formation, fetal development (folate)	carrots, oranges, bell peppers, mangoes, spinach, cantaloupes, butternut squash, Brussels sprouts, asparagus, avocados, tomatoes

NUTRIENT	SUPPORTS	PLANT-BASED SOURCES
VITAMIN B COMPLEX	cellular health, immune function, growth, red blood cell formation, energy levels, eyesight, brain function, healthy pregnancy, digestion, appetite, nerve function, heart health, hormonal health	nutritional yeast, whole grains, leafy greens, mangoes, carrots, sweet potatoes, sunflower seeds, legumes, peas, asparagus
VITAMIN C	healing from oxidative stress, immune function, collagen formation, iron absorption, wound healing, healthy skin, blood vessels, bones and cartilage	bell peppers, Brussels sprouts, citrus fruits, kiwis, tomatoes, broccoli, strawberries, spinach, cantaloupes, cauliflower
VITAMIN E	healing from oxidative stress, cellular protection, heart health, healthy vision, immune system, skin health, increased red blood cell count	sunflower seeds, avocado, broccoli, spinach, peanuts, almonds, tomatoes, leafy greens, pine nuts, butternut squash, soybeans

Our biggest concern when going plant-based was *will I get enough of what I need?* The answer is: yes, you can absolutely get what you need from plant sources.

We want to encourage you not to get too caught up in numbers, from counting calories to measuring macros. A better approach is to focus on eating enough calories and a variety of foods in an array of colors and let nature do the rest. **Focus on being calorie *conscious,* not calorie consumed!**

The beauty of a whole food, plant-based diet is that you can eat a high volume of food that's lower in calories and higher in nutrients—food freedom! You can eat an abundance, feel full and satiated, and actually be getting proper nourishment, all at the same time.

It's ideal if you can source local and seasonal produce, as it will contain the most nutrients and flavor. Furthermore, organic (which is automatically nonGMO), is going to be optimal. If you don't have access to organic or local, that doesn't mean don't eat it; the benefits of the plants will far outweigh any potential drawbacks.

Though we do not advocate for counting calories, tracking macros, or weighing meals, we do recommend checking out the Cronometer app to track your nutrient intake from time to time. It can help you determine which nutrients you may be getting too much of, or more important, not enough of.

As far as taking supplements go, we try to use them as a safeguard, not as a replacement for a well-rounded plant-based diet. The supplements that we take daily are:

- **Vitamin B$_{12}$**, which is the most important supplement on a plant-based diet. A common misconception is that B$_{12}$ is found in animal products; it is actually a bacteria found in the soil. This critical nutrient has been shown to be lacking in many vegetarian *and* nonvegetarian individuals. Many livestock are even given a B$_{12}$ supplement and dairy products are frequently fortified with it. We take a liquid B$_{12}$ sublingually (under the tongue) for optimal absorption.
- **Vitamin D$_3$**, which can also be obtained from safe levels of sun exposure
- **Omega-3 fatty acids**, including both of the two main types, EPA and DHA

It is best to get blood levels checked before supplementing, as it *is* possible to get *too much* of a good thing, which can lead to toxicity.

Note: While it is easy to get enough protein from whole food sources, we do incorporate protein powder into some of our smoothies and baked goods because we are highly active and athletic and enjoy the added boost of nutrition (and flavor). It is best to find a brand that is USDA organic and third-party tested. In our opinion, *clean* protein powder is an example of a "processed" or "refined" food with more benefits than drawbacks. Visit our "faves" page at EatMoveRest.com/Our-Faves for our brand recommendations.

The previous chart provides more on the benefits of these nutrients and other essential ones (regardless of your diet) with some suggestions for where to find them *in abundance* in plants, in the order we've found to be of most common concern.[9]

Eat the Rainbow

A colorful diet comes with a lot of perks. The benefits that plant foods impart can be identified by their color and a fair number of the associations are intuitive. For example, many red foods are good for your heart, and orange foods make your skin glow![10]

---

[9] Christian Koeder and Federico J. A. Perez-Cueto, "Vegan Nutrition: A Preliminary Guide for Health Professionals," *Critical Reviews in Food Science and Nutrition* 64, no. 3 (2024): 670–707, https://doi.org/10.1080/10408398.2022.2107997.

[10] Deanna M. Minich, "A Review of the Science of Colorful, Plant-Based Food and Practical Strategies for 'Eating the Rainbow,'" *Journal of Nutrition and Metabolism* (June 2019): 2125070, https://doi.org/10.1155/2019/2125070.

COLOR	SUPPORTS	PLANT-BASED SOURCES
RED	heart health, cell renewal, skin protection, cancer prevention, immune system	tomatoes, radishes, red cabbage, beets, red grapes, strawberries, watermelon, cherries, raspberries, pomegranates, cranberries, red apples
ORANGE AND YELLOW	immune system, eyesight, skin protection, healing from oxidative stress, heart health	carrots, pumpkin, sweet potatoes, yellow peppers, yellow tomatoes, mangoes, apricots, oranges, pineapples, oranges, grapefruit, peaches, papayas, pears
GREEN	detoxification, lower cholesterol, bone health, immune system, healthy eyesight, healthy pregnancy	broccoli, spinach, cabbage, green beans, zucchini, cucumbers, peas, green peppers, lettuce, Brussels sprouts, kale, kiwis, green apples, green grapes, lime, avocados
BLUE AND PURPLE	antiaging, heart health, memory, healthy blood vessels, gut health	eggplant, purple potatoes, blackberries, blueberries, purple grapes, plums, raisins, figs
WHITE	immune system, protection against viruses, lower cholesterol, liver detoxification	potatoes, onions, garlic, mushrooms, cauliflower, turnips, bananas, white nectarines, white peaches, pears

Troubleshooting

Here are some troubleshooting tips to help navigate allergies or sensitivities, digestive issues, or cravings on a plant-based diet. There are many different ways to do this lifestyle, so don't feel defeated! Also, be sure to join our online Eat Move Rest Club to connect with a community of like-minded individuals who are always eager to share new tips and strategies.

Allergies and Sensitivities

It's important to keep in mind that there is no diet of invincibility (but we do like our odds best on a whole foods, plant-based diet)! If you find that certain ingredients used in our recipes don't agree with you, here are some suggested alternatives so that you can enjoy the abundance of deliciousness in this book.

Nuts. In recipes that call for nuts or nut butter, try replacing them with seeds. Some good options are pumpkin, sunflower, hemp, chia, or flax, depending on what you're making. Some good nut-milk alternatives are coconut, rice, hemp, or oat milk.

Gluten. All recipes in this book can be prepared gluten-free, but if you are struggling with other recipes, our favorite gluten-free flour to use for baking is oat flour. We recommend avoiding bread altogether, as most gluten-free options are not nutritious. As for pasta, we love red lentil, brown rice, quinoa, and chickpea pastas.

Soy. In recipes that contain soybeans/edamame or tofu, you can either leave it out altogether or replace soybeans with lima beans or peas and replace tofu with white beans, chickpeas, or even black beans. Also be sure to try our homemade Red Lentil Tofu (page 117).

Grains. Replace grains such as brown rice with quinoa, millet, or amaranth, which are all actually seeds, not grains. You can also try sprouted whole grain and seed varieties, which are easier to digest.

Digestive Issues

When you start a new diet of any kind, your gut microbiome and digestive system will experience an acclimation period. Two common factors that could contribute to discomfort are: increased fiber intake and the order in which you consume various foods.

Fiber: We get a lot of questions about bloating, stomach cramps, sluggish digestion, and loose stools. The simplest answer is fiber. Fiber is not the enemy, though, it just takes your body time to acclimate, like anything new and unfamiliar. If you have to eat just one bean on day one, just eat one bean. On day two, two beans, and so on and so forth. It is also important to consume an adequate amount of both soluble and insoluble fiber. Soluble fiber attracts water and turns to a gel, which slows digestion. Examples include: nuts, seeds, beans, lentils, fruits, and many vegetables. Insoluble fiber is indigestible and adds bulk, helping to speed up digestion. Examples include: whole wheat and other whole grains and vegetables.

Beans: We love beans! They're one of the longevity foods most consumed by people living in the so-called Blue Zones of the world—where there is the highest concentration of centenarians. That being said, they have gotten a bad rap, and can cause some upset for certain individuals. When it comes to beans, rinse canned beans thoroughly. A better option would be to soak dry beans overnight (or at least six to eight hours) and then rinse and cook. This dramatically reduces any antinutrients and makes the nutrients more available to the body. Cooking from dry is the route that tends to agree more with peoples' guts! We like to use our pressure cooker to effortlessly (and quickly) cook our soaked dry beans without having to babysit them for two hours while they simmer on the stovetop. See our easy how-to on page 118.

Prebiotics and the Gut Microbiome: Prebiotics are indigestible, insoluble fiber that acts as food for the bacteria in your gut. If you're eating a wide variety of plant foods, you're helping to "seed" or "feed" your microbiome. The more you feed the beneficial bacteria in your gut flora, the more they proliferate—pretty cool, huh?! The scary thing is the same holds true for highly palatable, calorie-dense junk foods. The more you eat, the more you crave. There are actually more microbes (living organisms) in our gut than there are cells in our body, so we truly are what we eat! Even if you can't feel a positive difference immediately from eating nutrient-rich plant foods, your body is still shouting for joy at a cellular level. Eating high-prebiotic foods will lead to an overall healthier, happier, and better functioning gut.

Probiotics: Fiber-rich plant foods serve as prebiotic "food" for our probiotic gut flora, but you might also consider taking a probiotic supplement containing live strains of good bacteria and yeast to further support your microbiome. There are also many probiotic-rich foods such as sauerkraut, kimchi, tempeh, miso, and sourdough bread.

Hydration: We like to kick off our mornings with thirty-two ounces of fresh, filtered water. Hydration first thing in the morning will help to awaken your system and prepare your organs for digestion (a taxing task, believe it or not)!

Food Order: The way you are grouping your foods together could be another source of digestive distress. For example, it is best to eat melon by itself first thing in the morning as it is mostly water and highly digestible. If you eat a big, dense meal of cooked food and try to eat watermelon afterward, it will likely lead to stomach pain, bloating, and indigestion. While we don't suggest anyone adhere too rigidly to this formula, eating foods in the following order of digestibility might be beneficial if you are trying to heal your gut: filtered water, juice, smoothies, melon, other fruits, veggies and greens, and finally, cooked foods like starchy carbs, grains, beans, and legumes. Don't feel like you can't eat oatmeal for breakfast, though, but if you are in a state of distress, simplifying the flow of your foods in this way may help.

Cravings

The best way to overcome an unhealthy craving is to eliminate the temptation (don't bring junk foods into the house) and replace them with healthier alternatives. Do you constantly feel like you're fighting your sweet tooth? Stop fighting and start living! The best way to feel satisfied is to enjoy smoothies and fruits in abundance throughout the day, to satisfy your body's need for glucose from unrefined sources as fuel. This will help to cut down on refined sugar cravings. When you're really wanting something extra special, just treat yourself in the *right way*. The recipes in this book are free of refined sugar and other junk found in processed and packaged sweet treats. Many of the desserts are bite-size, making it easier to indulge and enjoy just enough to satisfy without going overboard. The Caramel Apple Cheesecake Bites (page 235) are out of this world! Medjool dates are another super simple, bite-size chewy treat. If a craving unexpectedly strikes, one or two of those usually does the trick. If something salty and/or crunchy is what you're craving, we've got options for that, too.

Plant-Based Pregnancy, Baby, and Child

Knowing another person's well-being depends on the diet and lifestyle choices that you make can be nerve-racking. Even if you're knowledgeable and have been eating a whole food, plant-based diet for a while, you may still find it a little scary to be responsible for knowing how to feed and nourish your kids the whole foods, plant-based way.

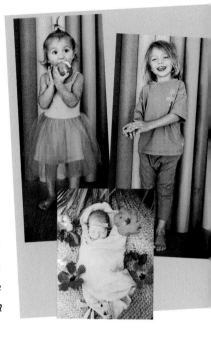

The good news is you're not the first parent to do it, and a wealth of science supports that a well-planned vegan diet is safe and beneficial for *all* stages of life, including pregnancy and infancy.[11] In fact, studies have found that vegan pregnant women have a lower-than-average rate of cesarean delivery, less postpartum depression, and lower neonatal and maternal mortality, with no complications or negative outcomes that are higher than average.[12] The key words here are *well-planned* (definitely!) and *vegan* (for us, a whole food, plant-based diet is the best option).

There are certainly some nutrients you'll want to pay extra-close attention to when it comes to pregnancy and nourishing small children, but the main thing to remember is abundance and variety.

Pregnancy and Postpartum

It's one thing to have your nutrition and fitness dialed in *before* children, but it's a whole new ball game when it comes to pregnancy and postpartum. I often get asked how I was able to "bounce back" after having two kids. The plain

[11]   G. B. Piccoli, R. Clari, F. N. Vigotti, F. Leone, R. Attini, G. Cabiddu, G. Mauro, N. Castelluccia, N. Colombi, I. Capizzi, A. Pani, T. Todros, and P. Avagnina, "Vegan-Vegetarian Diets in Pregnancy: Danger or Panacea? A Systematic Narrative Review," *BJOG: An International Journal of Obstetrics and Gynaecology* 122, no. 5 (April 2015): 623–33, https://doi.org/10.1111/1471-0528.1328012

[12]   F. Pistollato, S. Sumalla Cano, I. Elio, M. Masias Vergara, F. Giampieri, and M. Battino, "Plant-Based and Plant-Rich Diet Patterns During Gestation: Beneficial Effects and Possible Shortcomings," *Advances in Nutrition* 6, no. 5 (September 2015): 581–91, https://doi.org/10.3945/an.115.009126.

and simple answer is I never really had any bouncing back to do. Postpartum I experienced no pain and minimal discomfort, and after the "first forty days" spent resting, recovering, and moving at a slower pace with baby, I jumped right back into my exercise without a problem.

I think what helped me tremendously was having so much experience eating, moving, and resting my best beforehand. All too often, women become pregnant and decide it's time to get healthy or start exercising, and with morning sickness, nausea, aversions, and other "labor pains," it can be next to impossible to achieve those brand-new goals.

Now I know everybody, *every body*, is different, and each pregnancy, birth, and postpartum period is unique, and let me tell you, my journey didn't come without struggles, like the varicose veins, heartburn, slower digestion at times, and difficulty finding a comfortable position to sit or sleep in! The worst part was the nausea during the first trimester. They don't tell you that regardless of how healthy you are, there are some things you just can't escape—thanks hormones. So if you're struggling, know that it will pass, and you're not alone!

For a while during each pregnancy, I couldn't even look at anything leafy or green. I gave myself grace, listened to my body, and instead emphasized other healthy plant foods that were appealing to me—whole grains, beans, fruits, nutritious smoothies, and healthy fats. I guess you could say the weight gain was "all baby." Both children were born a healthy weight and length, breastfed well, and have been thriving ever since on a plant-based diet!

As for exercise, it was already built in to my morning routine, so nothing much changed there during pregnancy—in fact, I found it to be a much-needed reprieve from my nausea. I continued to exercise at the same intensity as before until I felt the need to modify and slow down and listened to my body just as I did with meals.

Pregnant and lactating women need more of just about everything, from vitamins and minerals to calories. It is of utmost importance to consume a wide variety of whole plant foods and to discuss taking a prenatal multivitamin with your health care provider, just to ensure your bases are covered. Opt for one derived from whole plant sources rather than a synthetic one (i.e., choose one that contains folate, not folic acid).

Protein, vitamin B_{12}, iron, zinc, iodine, omega-3 fatty acids, calcium, and vitamin D are important nutrients to stay on top of on a daily basis. Use the chart on pages 16–17 to see where to find them in abundance. Additionally, you'll want to make sure to get adequate folate, found in leafy greens, beans, and oranges.

Infancy and Childhood

For abundant milk supply and successful breastfeeding, my top tips are to:

- Stay properly hydrated with plenty of fresh filtered water and electrolytes.
- Get adequate calories from a variety of nutrient-dense plant foods.
- Experiment with galactagogues, which are certain foods that may boost milk supply. While studies are inconclusive, I can personally vouch for their effectiveness and have used oats, dates, chia seeds, flaxseeds, sweet potatoes, spinach, and brewer's yeast. Our Superfood Brownies (page 188) are loaded with galactagogues!

Baby-led weaning: We used the baby-led weaning approach for both kiddos, and it worked out wonderfully. It's a fuss-free way to introduce your baby to solid foods without having to mess with store-bought purees. Most of the time they can simply enjoy some form of whatever you're eating. You'll want to start with one, single whole food ingredient at a time. Soft is key! We recommend banana, avocado, or cooked sweet potato. After a few days, if your child hasn't experienced digestive distress or an allergic reaction, introduce one new food. It also gave me peace of mind to remember the phrase "under one, just for fun"

Did you know nearly all taste preferences are learned?

Infants begin to develop their taste preferences as early as fifteen weeks gestation. That means every single bite truly counts! Children continue to develop their taste preferences through breastmilk while breastfeeding.[13]

[13] Catherine A. Forestell, "Flavor Perception and Preference Development in Human Infants," *Annals of Nutrition and Metabolism* 70, suppl. no. 3 (2017): 17–25, https://doi.org/10.1159/000478759.

in regard to Baby experimenting with solid foods—don't sweat it too much if they're doing more finger painting than eating!

Nutrients of focus: When it comes to feeding babies, toddlers, and small children, it's important to place a bit more emphasis on healthy fats, plentiful protein, and iron-rich foods, on top of the other nutrients for all vegans mentioned in the Essential Nutrients and Potential Supplements section (pages 16–17). Healthy fat sources include avocados, nut and seed butters, and ground-up nuts and seeds in smoothies. Protein-rich foods also tend to be high in iron, and some great sources include beans, legumes, whole grains, soy, and leafy greens. Many of our kids' favorite meals and snacks in this book are noted with a (K).

Tips for Choosy Eaters

1. **Don't give up!** You may have to offer the same food thirty times before your choosy eater will finally try it—and like it! At mealtime, be sure to always include a "safe food" that you know your little one enjoys, so they begin to associate mealtime with a positive experience.
2. **Lead by example:** If you expect your little ones to eat whole plant foods, they've got to see you doing the same. Practice what you preach because as the saying goes, monkey see, monkey do!
3. **Engage and include:** Bring your kiddos grocery shopping with you and encourage them to choose their own fruits and vegetables and help prepare meals in the kitchen. Better yet, start a garden and let them help plant seeds, water sprouts, and eventually, harvest an abundance! Just remember to involve them in the three Ps, picking, planting, and prepping.
4. **Make meals fun:** Use chopped produce to make funny faces, rainbows, and other fun, vibrant designs on their plates. Give recipes fun names like Green Dino Smoothie (also known as our Go-To Green Protein Smoothie on page 81)! Easy-to-eat finger foods are always a safe bet, too. Lastly, simply offering the same foods in different ways might do the trick, like presenting them on a new pretty plate or instead of serving a bowl of oatmeal make baked oats (check out Baked Oats Two Ways on page 108).

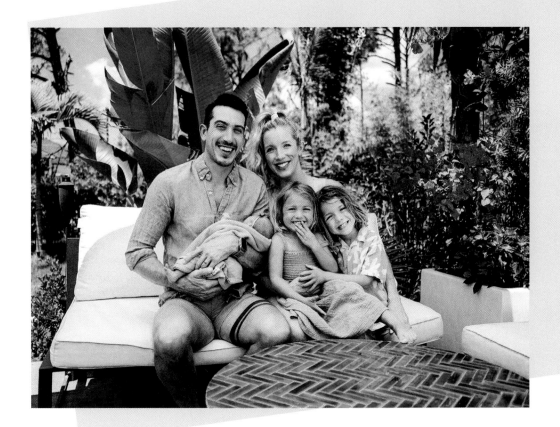

5. **Set boundaries:** Remind yourself it's only your job to decide *what* and *when* your children eat, and it's their job to decide *if* and *how much* they eat. Stand firm and continue offering healthy options for the whole family, and eventually choosy eaters palates will expand. Also remember to avoid yes or no answers by giving two options: *Would you like oatmeal or waffles for breakfast today?*

6. **Get creative:** To increase veggie consumption, try hiding foods like kale and cauliflower in colorful fruit smoothies. For a boost in calories, try adding avocados, nut/seed butters, hemp seeds, or coconut milk to sauces or smoothies.

MOVE

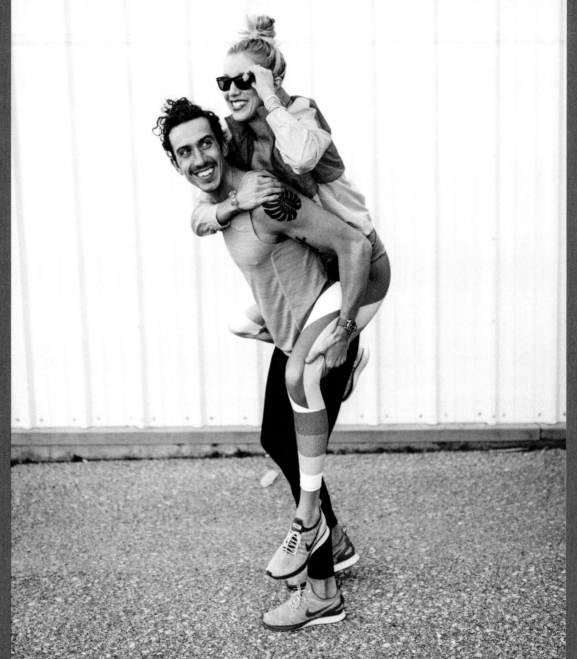

This is a big one for us—we *love* to move! For us, movement is not just essential to our daily lives, it's often the most *fun* part! We love creating guided workouts for our YouTube channel and daily fitness adventures for our Instagram stories. But it's not just fun. Daily activity plays an active role in our health and longevity.

Over two decades, Dan Buettner has studied the habits of people around the world who live beyond one hundred years old. Maybe you've read his book *The Blue Zones* or watched his *Live to 100* documentary on Netflix. In his research, Buettner frequently highlights the similarities in how long-lived people move their bodies. These folks, who are living to and beyond one hundred years old, didn't spend their twenties in the gym and aren't spending their later years there either. They aren't training hard for an hour and then sitting on their bums for the rest of the day. Instead, they participate in moderate movement *all day long.*

They walk to meet family or friends for morning coffee, ride their bikes to the market, and spend a couple of hours in the afternoon working in their gardens. In the evenings, they are on their feet preparing (healthy) food. These daily activities keep them nimble and their hearts pumping and their muscles strong.

While studies have shown that poor diet choices have the largest negative impact on health, there is plenty of evidence to suggest our less-active lives might also be contributing to poor health. You may have heard the frightening phrase "sitting is the new smoking." It may not be far off the mark. One of the leading experts on the benefits of exercise, Steven N. Blair, declared in a 2009 research paper that physical inactivity is the biggest public health problem of the twenty-first century.[1]

Dr. Michael Greger, who we've interviewed a few times on our YouTube channel, suggests that walking vegans are the healthiest. He recommends walking one hour a day, five days a week, but he also says the more the better. He shared that Japanese researchers concluded after a 2004 study on health practices and mortality that walking was so important, *not walking* is considered a "high risk

---

[1] Steven N. Blair, "Physical Inactivity: The Biggest Public Health Problem of the 21st Century," *British Journal of Sports Medicine* 43, no. 1 (January 2009): 1–2, https://bjsm.bmj.com/content/43/1/1

behavior" alongside smoking, excess alcohol consumption, and being obese.[2] So get those steps in!

While walking, stretching, and moving in general are critical for optimal health and longevity, we like to take our movement to the next level. Like Dr. Greger we think more is better.

Not only does regular movement support better physical health and positive body changes, it can boost your mood—almost instantly! Exercise has transformed our bodies and elevates our minds and moods on a daily basis.

Erin's Body Transformation Story

I started where most people start when they want to look better and feel better: exercise.

As a high school athlete with a personal trainer on the side, I was super active. I ran cross country for years and ran even more in the offseason just to stay in shape. I was also a varsity tennis player throughout high school, and that required me to stay strong and fit. I never had to worry about my weight. But as often happens, that all changed when the sports stopped and college started.

As I shared earlier, my early dorm days brought with them the "freshman fifteen," and then some. I felt "dense," both physically and mentally. When I decided to get healthy and start going to the campus recreation center, the first thing I did was step on the scale—big no-no! My heart sank. The number staring back at me was higher than I thought it ever would be. I fell into an all-too-common trap of self-loathing and finding approval of myself based on numbers on a scale or a clothing tag. I began riding the roller coaster of emotional highs and lows from "wow I look good in that picture" happiness to "my jeans don't fit anymore" distress. The good thing about all this is that it spurred me into action, and I began exercising like I knew how to from my high school days.

The more I went out, ate processed food, and stayed up late on the week-

---

[2] Y. Tsubono, Y. Koizumi, N. Nakaya, K. Fujita, H. Takahashi, A. Hozawa, Y. Suzuki, S. Kuriyama, I. Tsuji, A. Fukao, and S. Hisamichi, "Health Practices and Mortality in Japan: Combined Effects of Smoking, Drinking, Walking and Body Mass Index in the Miyagi Cohort Study," *Journal of Epidemiology* 14, suppl. no. 1 (February 2004): S39–45, https://doi.org/10.2188/jea.14.s39.

ends, the harder I would exercise during the week to "make up for it." While I did see results from exercise, I became burned out. I was overworked and underfed, but the number on the scale was going down, so I stuck with it thinking that results would equal more happiness and better health. I experienced neither.

I felt foggy in the afternoons, and I was always hungry but afraid to eat too much and gain more weight. Lean Cuisine and other packaged meals that advertised the promise of the perfect figure lured me in. But processed foods and my still unhealthy habits on the weekends kept me stuck. The roller coaster continued.

It wasn't until many years later that we realized you can't out-train a bad diet.

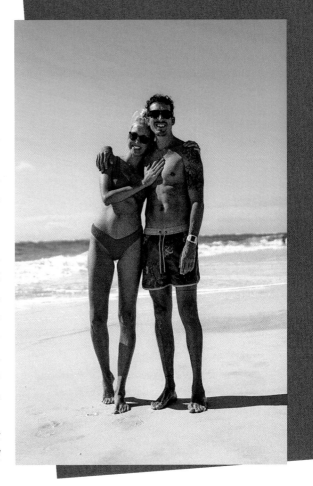

It wasn't until I began my plant-based journey that my health and happiness finally began to sync up. When I learned how to properly *nourish* my body, I no longer felt the need to *punish* myself with extreme workouts. This was a huge relief and led to even more progress in the gym and on my runs. My diet *fueled* my workouts.

I began to feel better and have more energy, and the excess weight started to melt off. I felt more aligned and less anxious. I began to shift my goals and my perspective from punishment to self-love and my focus from losing weight to building strength. I began to view exercise as a *moving meditation*, as it was a time to both clear my mind *and* allow my thoughts to flow freely.

My exercise routine went from painfully long runs, extreme forty-day HIIT challenges, and pricey gym memberships to forty-five-minute, easy-to-fit-in workout routines in our makeshift garage gym. I found a few free fitness influencers on social media who guided my sessions and kept me focused and encouraged. I started with a few dumbbells, adding more as I became stronger. I used to feel like I needed cardio to look and feel my best, but I've come to realize how beneficial and empowering resistance training is, especially since becoming a mom.

Personalize Exercise

The best place to start: **Do what "moves" you!**

We understand that some people, like my former Nebraska-football-playing brother, love pumping iron in the gym, while some prefer Sunday afternoon pickleball at the country club. What matters is getting it in. We often start by asking our coaching clients what *moves* them? Or what *used* to move them . . . Maybe they swam in high school, or like our endlessly romantic grandparents, maybe they often "went dancing." So, what is it for you?

If you like to dance, crank up the music and dance! If you have children, go outside and run around, throw a Frisbee, or kick a ball. If you like to be in nature, go for a walk or a hike. You get the idea. Doing what you already love to do is the best way to get the "ball rolling." Once you get a taste for how you feel after a good sweat session, not only will you *want* to make it a part of your daily routine, but you'll also look *forward* to it!

For those who struggle with exercise, Dusty likes to recommend making it an adventure. Start by taking the dog for an extra-long walk in a new part of your neighborhood. Make it fun for the both of you. Or go big and try an activity you've always wanted to pursue. Now might be the time to rent that kayak and get out on the water. Do what *moves* you!

Three Types of Movement

We like to focus on three types of movement: **cardiovascular, strength, and flexibility.** Finding a balance between these three types of physical activity is important for overall fitness. We both love cardio! Dusty likes to get out under the sun on his road bike, and I love my Peloton bike or a long run. Cardio gets your heart pumping, the sweat dripping, and it's not uncommon to experience what we have all heard of as "runner's high"!

Strength training has also been an important part of both our workout routines for years. We turned our garage into a gym years ago and started filling it with weights. We have a squat rack we also use for incline and bench press. We have a handful of dumbbells, pull-up bars, dip bars, and resistance bands, and even a weighted vest. While we typically have a lower heart rate and sweat less, strength training deserves all the credit for transforming our bodies. This is where fat is burned and muscles are made! Strength training also helps with bone density, which will help prevent injury as we age.

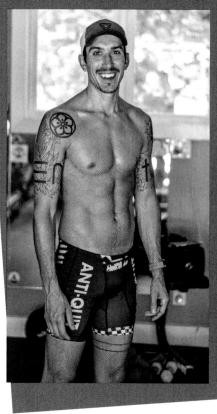

Finally, we improve our flexibility by stretching . . . every day! In fact, Dusty and Max share a bedtime stretching routine and make it part of their mindfulness and meditation time. Stretching keeps the muscles flexible, strong, and healthy, and we need that flexibility to maintain a range of motion in the joints. Without it, the muscles shorten and become tight. When you call on the muscles for activity, they are weak and unable to extend all the way, which puts you at risk for joint pain, strains, and muscle damage. The opposite is true of more flexible muscles—less pain, better range of motion, and more strength. The key with stretching is to do it often. The more you stretch, the more flexible you'll become.

Even when we travel, we can do all three forms of movement with *just* our bodies—no equipment needed! Cardio: go for a run. Strength: do push-ups, planks, and crunches. Flexibility: practice yoga and stretch as usual.

A combination of these three types of exercise will give you a stronger heart, lungs, muscles, and bones and maximum mobility for a long, healthy, and enjoyable life.

Here's a sample weekly workout. We exercise five to six days a week with one to two active recovery days, which include gentler forms of movement like a long walk or yoga.

Cardio: forty-five minutes, two to three times a week
- Aerobic or "cardio" activities make your heart beat faster and make you breathe harder. They strengthen your heart and lungs and build up your endurance.
  - brisk walking
  - cycling
  - running

Strength: forty-five to sixty minutes three times a week
- Strength or resistance training activities make your muscles work against, or "resist," something, which helps tone and strengthen your muscles and bones.
  - lifting weights
  - body-weight exercises like doing push-ups or pull-ups

Stretching: fifteen to twenty minutes every day (ideally when the muscles are warmed up)
- Stretching helps with range of motion, flexibility, and recovery.
  - touching toes
  - using a foam roller
  - practicing yoga

Sometimes cardio and strength training will overlap, like during a sweaty HIIT or circuit workout, and sometimes we'll divide time equally between a twenty-five-minute cardio run/ride and a twenty-five-minute lift.

Our Top Five Ways to Move

1. **Cycling:** We both do more cycling than anything. Cycling is nice because you can do it inside on a stationary bike or outside. It's great for both be-

ginners or advanced athletes. It is also very low impact, which makes it a lifelong sport and easier for those who may be dealing with past injuries to the back or joints.

Starting out tip: Try a friends or family ride at a "conversational" pace before breaking out the spandex.

2. **Running**: We like running for its full-body benefits and because it only requires a supportive pair of running shoes. Because it is higher impact, it builds strong muscles and bones. Depending on your fitness level, you can run faster and for longer distances, or work your way up from brisk walking to a jog.

Starting out tip: Try intervals. Walk for two minutes then run for two minutes, rotating for twenty minutes, total.

3. **Calisthenics:** Body-weight training is nice because it doesn't require a gym or a lot of equipment. Some of the fittest people we follow are body-weight-only trainers who focus on military-style exercises that can be done anywhere.

Starting out tip: Do push-ups, sit-ups, squats, and lunges in your living room.

4. **Machine and free-weight training:** To build lean muscle tissue, you have to use more resistance than your muscles are used to, which over time will increase your strength. While calisthenics are great, some people will have more success using free weights or resistance machines.

Starting out tip: Most gyms offer free trial periods and even a free session with a personal trainer who can help you assess what type of resistance training is right for you.

5. **Sports:** Tennis anyone? How about a pickup basketball game or sand volleyball tournament? Sports are great because they make movement fun! Competition is also a good motivator.

Starting out tip: Try pickleball! It's super popular right now and is great for all ages and fitness levels.

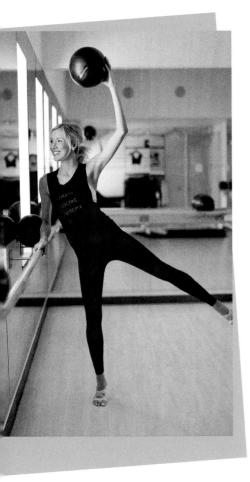

Motivation, Goal Setting, and Consistency

Motivation

The best way to stay motivated is to find a form of movement you enjoy. If you don't enjoy what you're doing, motivation will quickly fade. Then pair that up with a goal. Motivation is a reward-based system in human beings, meaning, to feel motivated, there needs to be a goal or purpose in place and a benefit we get as a result of achieving it. For example, your goal could be to finish a run, and that sense of accomplishment plus the rush of endorphins motivates you to do it again the next day. Or your goal could be to be able to do a strength-training workout with fifteen-pound weights and, once you accomplish it, see the visible results in your before-and-after photos, which encourages you to set a new lifting goal. These incremental successes fuel us to keep going.

Goal Setting

Just like getting in your car in the morning, it's important to know where you're going. If you didn't, you would literally be wasting time and fuel. The same is true for your fitness. Without a clear destination in mind, you will just be burning time and energy. Some might consider that enough, but we can assure you, you will have more success if you start by setting some simple goals for yourself.

Steps
- Identify the result you'd like to achieve.
- Work backward from the end goal, creating benchmarks.
- Make benchmarks realistic and attainable.
- Make them trackable (time, distance, etc.).
- Reward yourself every time you reach a new benchmark.

Example

Goal: Run a 5k by the end of the month

Benchmarks: Week 1: walk/run 1k. Week 2: walk/run 3k. Week 3: 3k, no walking. Week 4: run 1k every day. End of week 4: run 5k!

Reward: for every completed benchmark I get to _____.

Consistency Is KEY!

To achieve a desired goal, you need to work toward it regularly. This is true for every goal or outcome you wish to achieve. Doing something consistently and not just when you feel inspired and motivated to do it, isn't just important, it's necessary.

Consistency means focusing on the task at hand while still maintaining a long-term vision. When we do something regularly, we get feedback that helps us change course when required.

In other words, consistency is all about repetition. It's about repeating the same actions, habits, and rituals, day in and day out, gaining feedback from these actions, and adjusting them accordingly to help stay on track as we work toward our goal. The cool thing is, that feedback we receive will in most cases be positive. Positive reinforcement, like reaching your run goal, makes you feel good, which increases motivation and makes consistency *easy!*

Starting out tip: find an accountability partner, join a group, or hire a trainer. We are much more likely to succeed when we have other people counting on us!

The best part about consistency and moving regularly are the results. A year from now, you will be glad you started today! At the end of the day, you'll likely experience an improved quality of sleep thanks to getting in some movement, and quality rest also equals quality repairs. It's a win-win!

REST

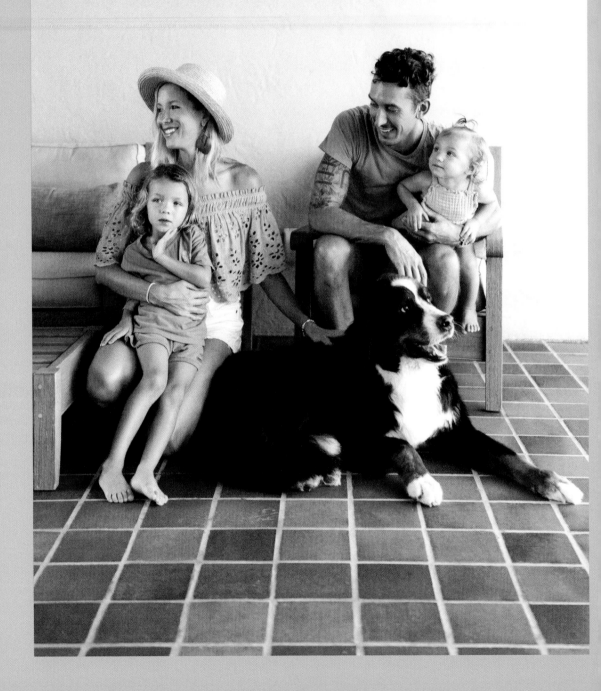

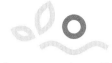 Rest—the third and final piece of the "back to the basics" puzzle—is often undervalued, but research confirms how important it really is.

"There will be sleeping enough in the grave." This famous quote often attributed to Benjamin Franklin, among others, is wrong. Science has shown undeniably that rest, and sleep in particular, is essential to our health and longevity.

Sleep is restorative, giving our cells the chance to repair and our muscles to recover. You can't make gains in the gym without proper rest, and sleep deprivation or disrupted sleep is associated with an increased risk of developing depression and anxiety, hypertension, cancer, and other health conditions.[1] We all know that we just don't feel our best or function well without a good night's rest. On top of that, when you haven't gotten adequate sleep, the two hunger hormones, leptin and ghrelin, go into overdrive, making you more susceptible to bingeing and indulging in cravings.

Okay, you all get it. Sleep (around eight hours) is important. But what about "rest"?

Our Definition of "Rest"

We like to say that rest is often what comes after Eat and Move. . . . It's "the rest." Sleep is included but so is taking time to simply breathe, stretch, kick back with a book, meditate, journal, pray, worship, or spend some quality downtime with your family and friends. It's the "wind-down and charge-up" time.

It sounds easy, but rest can be hard! Who has the time?

We are living in an age where we get rewarded for the hustle. If we aren't working, we should be. We are constantly bombarded with information, always learning, always entertained, *always connected*. We are busier than ever.

We also don't get rewarded for rest like we do for eating well or cranking out a 6 a.m. sweat session. No one is posting selfies of themselves "in bed early

---

[1]   Adam J. Krause, Eti Ben Simon, Bryce A. Mander, Stephanie M. Greer, Jared M. Saletin, Andrea N. Goldstein-Piekarski, and Matthew P. Walker, "The Sleep-Deprived Human Brain," *Nature Reviews Neuroscience* 18, no. 7 (2017): 404–18, https://doi.org/10.1038/nrn.2017.55.

tonight" or "waking up after a full nine hours," right? It's as if resting is a sign of weakness and we are made to feel guilty for needing it.

But here's the thing. If we *do* rest better, we will also do everything *else* better.

Remember during a preflight safety check when the flight attendant says, "In case of emergency, place your oxygen mask on before assisting others"? That is because if you pass out, you're not going to be able to help anyone else. The same is true of rest. If you don't do it for you, you won't be able to do the other things in life that are important, so get your rest!

We like to use the seven types of rest Dr. Saundra Dalton-Smith describes in her book *Sacred Rest* to identify the various kinds of activities that should be considered rest:

1. **Physical rest:** divided into passive forms such as sleeping/napping and active forms such as stretching, leisure walks, and massage therapy to help improve circulation in the body
2. **Mental rest:** quieting your thought process and clearing your mind for better focus and clarity
3. **Emotional rest:** practicing authenticity and vulnerability by expressing your feelings with people you trust
4. **Spiritual rest:** focusing on building an intimate relationship with God over ritualistic religious routines
5. **Social rest:** spending time with people who do not put any demands on you and simply enjoy being with you
6. **Sensory rest:** downgrading the external sensory input from your electronics as well as the lights and sounds in your environment.
7. **Creative rest:** allowing yourself opportunities to appreciate natural beauty (the beach, flowers) or man-made beauty such as artwork, and letting it inspire creativity inside yourself

Buzz Word: Meditation

Has anyone else felt pressured to adopt a meditation practice lately? I think we all probably have. "Meditation" is definitely having a moment right now, but for most of us, meditation is not something that comes easily—and that's all the more reason to practice it! Okay, but why?

We've found that meditation has helped increase and amplify our positive emotions. It has also helped improve our focus and therefore productivity and creativity.

Maybe you're familiar with the term *looking-glass self.* The looking-glass self was first coined by Charles Cooley, and it describes how our own identity is dependent upon our perceived appearance by others. Crazy. Sad. We are who we think other people think we are. We need to shift focus and step into our own authenticity, separate from how we think the world sees us; we do this through quiet, focused self-observation, aka meditation.

Meditation has improved our relationship with each other, our kids, our families, and most important, with ourselves. It is a powerful, and, we think, necessary tool for cultivating and nurturing creativity, spirituality, peace, love, joy, and change.

Meditation can take many different forms. It can mean sitting quietly, eyes closed, or it can be a "moving" meditation such as a good long run or bike ride. When the body begins to move, the mind begins to move, too. Whenever Erin falls into a rut or a pattern of "stinking thinking" as our mentor Joel Christiansen says, she laces up and hits the pavement.

Dusty's meditation practice is every night for about fifteen to twenty minutes before bed. He, and often Max, too, spends this time quietly stretching and breathing in an almost pitch-black room. It's rarely silent between farts, giggles, and the never-ending stream of four-year-old questions, but it works.

All that being said, meditation can and does often "work" best through silence and stillness. Peace and quiet was a lot easier to come by before kids, but finding calm amid the chaos is when our "practice" is truly put to the test and begins to deepen! We only become stronger in a skill when faced with a bit of resistance or "heavy lifting." We find it helpful to use the following techniques to focus the mind:

- **Memorization:** Reciting a quote, verse, or prayer with an uplifting message can help to calm the mind and boost the spirit. This can be especially helpful in states of distress when it's difficult to put your own thoughts into words. Autopilot via memorization can help to direct the mind, soften the noise, and calm the chaos.
- **The breath:** Try box breathing. Inhale for a count of seven seconds, hold at the top for seven, exhale for seven, hold at the bottom for seven, and repeat. You can also try breathing in for four seconds and out for seven seconds. Breath work can help to slow the heart rate and steady the mind.
- **Visualization:** Successful athletes visualize victory, and you can do the same. Focus on where you see yourself in five, ten, or fifteen years or a goal you'd like to achieve. You can also visualize a past experience that brought you joy, such as a memorable vacation, a fun time with friends, your wedding day, or the birth of a child.
- **The body:** Try doing a full-body scan, beginning at the toes and working your way up to the crown of the head. Focus on each and every muscle group, limb, digit, and organ. Try not to get caught up in any pain or discomfort you might feel. Instead, just notice it, and move on. You can also focus on the senses: sight, sound, taste, touch, and smell.

Now as a mom of three, Erin rarely finds much space or silence for a sweetly serene meditation practice, but she still tries to take moments to slow down and get focused again. Life is messy, and rarely perfect, so she reminds herself that it's most important to do her best to remain in a meditative state throughout all her daily doings. That's where mindfulness comes in. . . .

The Eat Move Rest Tool Chest
Head to our YouTube channel for a beginner ten-minute meditation that encompasses all these techniques!

Mindfulness

We define mindfulness as becoming more aware of and, more important, staying in the present moment. We both began to practice mindfulness after having kids. As a result, we both have seen a reduction in stress, anxiety, and even depressing thoughts. We've had therapists say anxiety comes from future-tripping, and depression comes from dwelling in the past, so the antidote to both is staying in the present moment. The way we do that is by practicing mindfulness and intentionality.

Our mindfulness practices have helped slow our reaction time in stressful situations, particularly with the kids. Instead of responding to outbursts with our own, being mindful helps us to pause, take a deep breath, and think about how we ought to respond, and therefore do it better.

Social scientists say that children learn more from the types of behavior they *see* rather than what they are *told*. Instead of yelling, lecturing, or talking, we stay quiet and mindful, and we show them how to be in the world by modeling the behavior we'd like to see.

When it comes to food, mindfulness can be as easy as taking a moment to:

- bless your meal or offer up gratitude for it;
- focus on your breath to slow down and prepare your mind for what you're about to eat;
- ask, "Is what I'm about to eat going to help me or hinder me?";
- visualize where the food on your plate came from and who cultivated it, picked it, shipped it, and prepared it; and
- become aware of how the food on your plate is fueling your body—from the tiniest cell to the largest organ.

A Mindful Morning and Evening Routine

Let's face it, our minds are very "full," but that's okay! Being mindful helps make sense and order out of a messy monkey mind. Mindfulness has been so hugely important for accomplishing tasks and reaching goals in our lives. Even before we wake up in the morning, we're practicing mindfulness the night before.

We like to make a list or a road map of where we'd like the day to go. A typical road map looks like this:

- exercise/movement
- educational activity w/ kids
- social media post
- content creation (YouTube shoot)
- coaching call
- brand call
- check emails
- write/blog
- edit/prepare content

This daily road map is sandwiched between a morning and/or evening routine that focuses on self-care. Here's an example of an ideal morning and evening routine for us:

Morning
- prayer, read devotional or Scripture
- step outside on the grass and watch the sun rise
- meditation, breath work, and stretching
- make the bed, brush teeth, get everyone dressed
- hydrate (tall glass of filtered water)
- fuel up (smoothie and/or juice)

Evening
- play, get outside with the kids
- prepare a nourishing dinner
- pray and eat as a family
- clean up, shower, skincare routine
- watch a movie, read, or play
- pray, make tomorrow's list, and go to bed

Even just picking one or two of these to do each day can be super beneficial. If you alternate, then you won't tire of doing the exact same thing each and every day. For example, maybe one day you feel more drawn to journaling than meditation, and the next day, maybe you only have time for an "internal journal" session (a mental gratitude check-in), and the next day, you really just want to dive into a spiritual text.

Rest and mindfulness practices come in many forms, and consistency simply means showing up in some way (not necessarily in the same way) to nurture your soul every day, just like it's healthy to vary your fitness regimen and diet.

Going "Beyond the Plate": Building and Nurturing a Relationship with God

Eating well is not only important but necessary for good health and longevity. Exercise and daily movement is also an esteemable act. Every time we sweat, it boosts our spirits, energy increases, mental clarity improves, and sleep gets better, too. But when we started posting content, the feedback we received and the types of people we were attracting all had very common traits, and it wasn't just about food.

We often found ourselves moving "beyond the plate" and into conversations and interactions around spirituality, entertaining questions like "What's the meaning of all this?"

1 Corinthians 6:19 says, "Do you not know that your bodies are temples of the Holy Spirit, who is in you, whom you have received from God? You are not your own." This encourages us to take care of our temples by eating, moving, and resting our best, for sure. It also reminds us that we are *spiritual* beings having a *human* experience.

Our retreat participants, those who've decided to take the next steps toward life-transforming change, come in search of more than a smoothie recipe or workout routine—they come for greater healing. Healing of the heart must take place beyond weight loss.

Brian and Jody Calvi—our longtime friends and owners of Finca de Vida, the retreat center we attend in Costa Rica—are great facilitators when it comes to all forms of healing, but one thing they always focus on is forgiveness.

While food may be the portal to better health and what often brings us together, it is love and forgiveness that pave the path to ultimate healing and radical transformation.

So how do we grow in love, find spirituality, and foster forgiveness both within ourselves and with others?

We believe transformation begins with entertaining the idea that we are children of an all-loving and forgiving Creator. Whether you choose to acknowledge this relationship by spending time in nature and feeling gratitude for all of God's creations, attending church services, reading Scripture, or praying at home, you are strengthening your spiritual life.

There is a saying that goes "I'd rather spend time on a mountain thinking about God, than spend time in a church thinking about a mountain." Do what you feel brings you in closest connection to our Creator—we acknowledge that there are many perspectives on this. As the saying goes, the ocean can look very different depending on whether you're swimming below its waters, standing on its shore, or soaring above it in a plane, and yet the ocean is the same. The important factor is cultivating that relationship with our divine Creator.

We come sharing, as the saying goes, not from the mountaintop but from the mud; not as spiritual guides or leaders, but as fellow explorers.

We have come to recognize not just the benefit but the necessity of cultivating a spiritual practice as a form of *soul food*.

We sometimes say that God is like our built-in GPS, always guiding and rerouting us when we inevitably make a wrong turn.

Try this: when you wake up tomorrow morning, before you start to think about your first meal or your workout, try to consider how you can first fulfill your spiritual quota, and be present and aware throughout your day, as well.

An Open Mind and the Power of Visualization

Keeping an open mind is important in life but especially when you are thinking about making a change. We tend to stick to our familiar habits and practices even if we realize they're not working for us—and there ends all opportunity for growth.

Don't let that be you. The ideas and information in this book may be new or challenging to you. Allow us to offer you a temporary "learner's permit" or even just an "observer's permit" to help you keep an open mind.

If you allow the practices and recipes in this book to sink in, you may find they start to make sense and transform your life as they have ours.

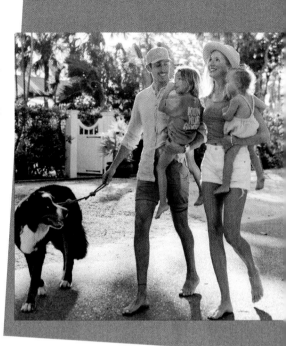

Transformation will take action! We must have faith in our abilities to try something new and visualize ourselves succeeding.

Visualization is powerful because it's been shown to trick the brain into believing the vision is real. In one famous experiment conducted by neurologist Alvaro Pascual-Leone, volunteers from one group were asked to play a simple sequence of piano notes each day for five consecutive days, after which their brains were scanned (each day) in the region connected to the finger muscles. Another set of volunteers were asked to *imagine* playing the same notes instead, also having their brains scanned each day. Results showed the changes in the brain in those who *imagined* playing the piano were the same as in those who *actually* played piano.[2] Incredible!

The unknown can be frightening, but only if you see failure on the other side of that fear. What if on the other side of that fear, we visualize ourselves succeeding, growing, or at the very least, learning?

We encourage you to dream big! Visualize a world and a life you would love to live and start creating it. Reinforce that image of yourself through habits that support eating, moving, and resting your best!

Erin recently took a white marker and wrote empowering messages on every mirror in our house: "You are awesome!," "I'm perfect!," and "Be-you-tiful!" It seemed cheesy at first, but once we committed to seeing ourselves in a positive light, we started becoming that positive version of ourselves.

Do you see yourself as you always have been? Could you see yourself as who you would like to become? The good news: you get to choose, starting now!

Let's go!

---

2   A. Pascual-Leone, D. Nguyet, L. G. Cohen, J. P. Brasil-Neto, A. Cammarota, and M. Hallett, "Modulation of Muscle Responses Evoked by Transcranial Magnetic Stimulation During the Acquisition of New Fine Motor Skills," *Journal of Neurophysiology* 74, no. 3 (September 1995): 1037–45, https://doi.org/10.1152/jn.1995.74.3.1037.

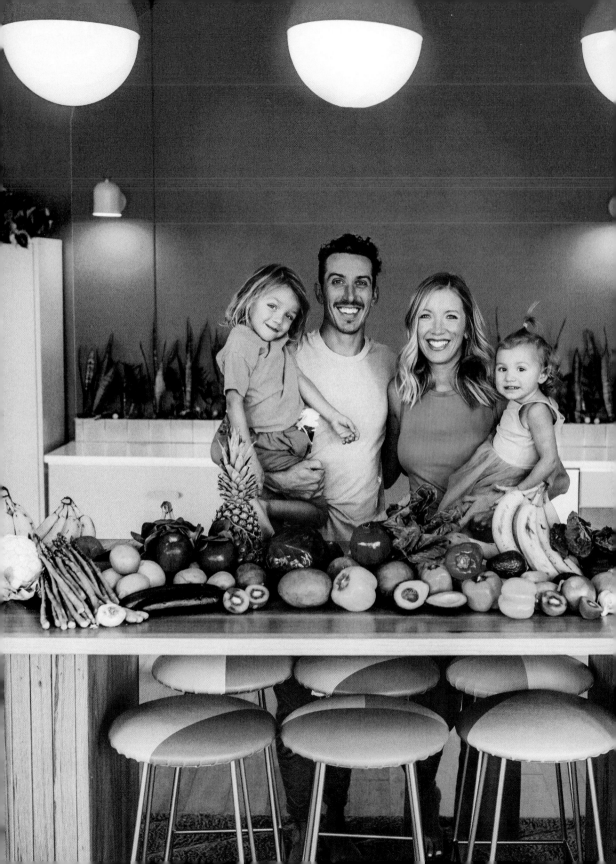

Part Two
Eat Move Rest: Meal, Movement & Mindfulness Plan

(more than just a meal plan)!

This is where *you* get to put Eat Move Rest to the test and find out how much it can do for you. We started *our* plant-based journey with a forty-day challenge, and it felt like the perfect length of time to really get the hang of things and feel our best. The number forty also has great symbolic meaning.

The number forty signifies new life, growth, and transformation. The human gestation period is forty weeks, the postpartum "first forty days" is a sacred period of bonding and restoration, the Israelites wandered in the desert for forty years, Jesus fasted for forty days.... You get the idea.

During and after completing this forty-day plan, you'll experience the following benefits:

- improved mental clarity
- weight optimization
- more energy
- better digestion
- clearer skin

- deeper sleep
- lower stress and anxiety
- self-empowerment
- and so much more!

That said, it is also common to experience some detox symptoms such as headaches, nausea, bloating, or other digestive issues depending on your current diet and lifestyle. This is your body clearing out the junk! These physical symptoms will pass. Try to stay committed and power through but also listen to your body and, as always, consult with your health care practitioner before making any diet or lifestyle changes.

Make this plan the first step on your journey to recover your health and happiness—and give you the oomph you need to get you from where you are currently to where you want to be. Becoming your best self truly starts by doing the three things we all do every day, *better!*

Here's how the next forty days will unfold:

- Days 1–10 introduce whole food, plant-based meals
- Days 11–20 add on movement
- Days 21–30 add on mindfulness
- Days 31–40 empower you to create your own plan, combining meals, movement, and mindfulness!

Get Ready

Prepare yourself for the next forty days by getting into the right mindset. Try any or all of these options:

- Focus on the number forty and what it symbolizes.
- Share your goals and plan with others for accountability.
- Practice positivity. You can do this!
- Write empowering words or quotes on sticky notes and place them throughout your home.
- Begin a gratitude journal.
- Experiment with visualization. Close your eyes and envision yourself succeeding and imagine how good you're going to feel afterward.
- Last but not least, get excited and own this journey!

Meals: Days 1 to 10

We handpicked some of our most tried-and-true recipes that have been with us since the beginning. Not only are they family favorites, they're also beginner-friendly, super tasty, and hyper-nourishing, to give you the best possible benefit during this challenge.

You can expect breakfasts filled with nutrient-dense smoothies, fresh fruit, and oatmeal, lunches loaded with rainbow-licious salads, and dinners with hearty and warming, protein-packed soups, curries, stews, and so much more. Find your favorites and get used to them, and when you're ready, begin creating your own versions of each recipe!

Prep

Review the recipes for the next ten days (all the recipes are in this book), make a grocery list, and do your shopping run: stock up on fruits, veggies, whole grains, nuts, and seeds!

Prep as much as possible early in the week to help make mealtime less stressful and more streamlined. Our top tips include the following:

- Freeze smoothie ingredients in reusable, sealable storage bags so they are ready to dump into your high-speed blender and blend in the morning.
- Juice extra ginger and/or turmeric and freeze in ice cube trays to pop into smoothies.
- Soak dry beans and cook them in a pressure cooker for the easiest, hands-off prep. (See directions on page 118.)
- Cook a large batch of grains and/or legumes (quinoa, brown rice, lentils).
- Prepare homemade plant milk, hummus, salsa, and/or dressings.
- Make a batch of Strawberry Banana Muffins (page 191) or Caramel Delight Cookies (page 232) so you have those snacks at the ready.
- Rinse and dry fresh fruit. Chop and add to containers.
- Chop veggie sticks and add to containers.

EAT	BREAKFAST	LUNCH	SNACK	DINNER
Day 1	Go-To Green Protein Smoothie (page 81) + piece of fruit	Veggie-ful Breakfast Scramble (page 100)	veggies + Creamy Cashew Cheeze dip (page 219), Homestyle Hummus (page 213), or Grateful Green Guacamole (page 215)	Root Veggie Stew (page 158)
Day 2	Flip-Free Protein Pancakes (page 107) or Banana Oat Waffles (page 104)	Fiesta Color Wheel Salad (page 123)	Fantastic Fruit Plate (page 97) and/or Banana Sushi (page 187)	Root Veggie Stew (leftover)
Day 3	Flip-Free Protein Pancakes or Banana Oat Waffles (leftover)	Build Your Own Açaí or Pitaya Smoothie Bowl (page 90)	1–2 Strawberry Banana Muffins (page 191)	Rainbow Mango Pad Thai (page 120)
Day 4	Green Machine Detox Juice (page 63) + fresh fruit of choice	Better-for-You Burrito Balance Bowl (page 116)	Fantastic Fruit Plate (page 97) and/or Vanilla Bean Overnight Oats (page 111)	Bountiful Black Bean Veggie Burgers (page 141)
Day 5	Wild Blueberry Detox Green Smoothie (page 83) + Fantastic Fruit Plate (page 97)	Pineapple (Un)fried Rice (page 128)	1–2 Strawberry Banana Muffins (leftover)	Build Your Own Balance Bowl (page 119) + Bountiful Black Bean Veggie Burgers (leftover)
Day 6	Sweet Green Energy Juice (page 64)	Pineapple (Un)fried Rice (leftover)	1–3 Caramel Delight Cookies (page 232)	Coconut Quinoa Yellow Curry (page 148)
Day 7	Go-To Green Protein Smoothie (page 81) + piece of fruit	Colorful Collard Wraps (page 138)	veggies + Creamy Cashew Cheeze dip (page 219), Homestyle Hummus (page 213), or Grateful Green Guacamole (page 215)	Coconut Quinoa Yellow Curry (leftover)
Day 8	Green Machine Detox Juice (page 63) + fresh fruit of choice	Superseed Everything Salad (page 124)	Tangerine Dream Immunity Smoothie (page 86)	Chickpea Falafel Patties (page 142)
Day 9	Apple Banana Date Porridge (page 103)	Superseed Everything Salad (leftover)	1–3 Caramel Delight Cookies (page 232)	Build Your Own Balance Bowl (page 119) + Chickpea Falafel Patties (leftover)
Day 10	Un-Beetable Preworkout Smoothie (page 85)	Butternut Squash Pomegranate Quinoa Salad (page 131)	Fantastic Fruit Plate (page 97)	Sweet Potato and Kale Chili (page 156)

Movement: Days 11 to 20

Continue following the Days 1 to 10 meal plan, or if you're feeling ready for it, select your own meals from the other recipes in this book. Make sure you are properly fueled and hydrated before exercise!

Now, let's get moving! Over the next ten days, you'll add daily exercise. In order to assess whether the beginner, intermediate, or advanced exercise option is best for you, consider:

- How often do you currently exercise? If you don't exercise at all, the beginner level might be best for you. If you are familiar with various forms of fitness but aren't exercising as consistently as you'd like, the intermediate approach might be a good fit. If you exercise regularly and want to challenge yourself, go for the advanced!
- Do you have any injuries or physical limitations? If yes, first consult with your health care practitioner to okay any new form of fitness. Identify for yourself which types of movement feel best to you. Remember, exercise shouldn't hurt your joints or create strain, but you may experience discomfort in the form of muscle fatigue and shortness of breath during cardio—this is your chance to experience new challenges and growth!

"Bonus" exercises are perfect to do in the evening before winding down for bed or first thing in the morning. Any fitness level can do the bonus!

The following plan was designed to encompass the three main areas of fitness: strength, cardio, and flexibility. You can find free guided workouts to fit into this program either on our YouTube channel or others, or simply guide yourself if you are experienced.

Prep

For your ten days of movement, the following tools can be helpful, but are not required:

- shoes with good support for walking, running, biking, etc.
- yoga mat or soft surface for stretching and yoga
- light (5 lb.), medium (10 to 15 lb.), and heavy dumbbells (15 to 25 lb.) for resistance training

- resistance bands for sculpting and toning
- bike or stationary bike for a cardio alternative to running
- access to YouTube/internet for free workouts (our Eat Move Rest channel and others)

We are all in different seasons of life and at different levels of fitness, so do what works for you. Know your limits—kick your ego to the curb and give yourself grace in the process. At the same time, remember how it feels to cut corners (not good). You get out what you put in, so really give it your all. A thirty- or sixty-minute sweat session is such a small fraction of your twenty-four-hour day, but it can have a profound and long-lasting positive impact on your physical and mental well-being.

MOVE	BEGIN-NER	INTERMEDIATE	ADVANCED	BONUS
DAY 11	walk, jog, or yoga for 30 min.	HIIT or circuit workout w/ dumbbells (full body) 30 min.	HIIT or circuit workout w/ dumbbells (full body) 45 min.	10-min. walk, stretch, or yoga
DAY 12	walk, jog, or yoga for 30 min.	HIIT or circuit workout w/ dumbbells (full body) 30 min.	HIIT or circuit workout w/ dumbbells (full body) 45 min.	10-min. walk, stretch, or yoga
DAY 13	walk, jog, or yoga for 30 min.	cardio 15 min. (run, ride, row, etc.) + yoga 15 min.	cardio 25 min. (run, ride, row, etc.) + yoga 20 min.	10-min. walk, stretch, or yoga
DAY 14	walk, jog, or yoga for 30 min.	HIIT or circuit workout w/ dumbbells (full body) 30 min.	HIIT or circuit workout w/ dumbbells (full body) 45 min.	10-min. walk, stretch, or yoga
DAY 15	walk, jog, or yoga for 30 min.	HIIT or circuit workout w/ dumbbells (full body) 30 min.	HIIT or circuit workout w/ body weight (full body) 45 min.	10-min. walk, stretch, or yoga
DAY 16	walk, jog, or yoga for 30 min.	cardio 15 min. (run, ride, row, etc.) + yoga 15 min.	HIIT or circuit workout w/ dumbbells (full body) 45 min.	10-min. walk, stretch, or yoga

Day 17	walk, jog, or yoga for 30 min.	HIIT or circuit workout w/ dumbbells (full body) 30 min.	cardio 25 min. (run, ride, row, etc.) + yoga 20 min.	10-min. walk, stretch, or yoga
Day 18	walk, jog, or yoga for 30 min.	HIIT or circuit workout w/ dumbbells (full body) 30 min.	HIIT or circuit workout w/ dumbbells (full body) 45 min.	10-min. walk, stretch, or yoga
Day 19	walk, jog, or yoga for 30 min.	cardio 15 min. (run, ride, row, etc.) + yoga 15 min.	HIIT or circuit workout w/ dumbbells (full body) 45 min.	10-min. walk, stretch, or yoga
DAY 20	walk, jog, or yoga for 30 min.	HIIT circuit workout w/ dumbbells (full body) 30 min.	cardio 25 min. (run, ride, row, etc) + Yoga 20 min.	10 min walk, stretch, or yoga

Mindfulness: Days 21 to 30

Continue eating plant-powered meals and moving daily. If you did the intermediate exercise option, consider trying the advanced, or if you haven't already, try adding in the bonus routine each day.

Mindfulness can take many forms. Meditation is the seemingly most common but also the most difficult! Relax. We included quiet meditation as part of the plan but also some other forms of mindfulness to give you a sampling.

We have found that repetitive morning and evening routines can lose their luster and drive us into autopilot where we almost forget why we're doing what we're doing. Instead, simply incorporating *some* type of mindfulness each day can be more engaging and fulfilling. That's why we've included three options for each day. Pen to paper, reading and reflecting, deep and meaningful conversation, time in nature, and creative movement all have a place here. Enjoy the variety and take note of what moves (or stills) you most. This just might be the portal into greater understanding of yourself and how to make friends with your mind!

Prep

For your ten days of mindfulness, the following tools can be helpful, but are not required:

- a journal to write down your thoughts and goals
- headphones for listening to guided meditations

- guided-meditation app or access to YouTube/internet for free content
- devotional book of your choice
- white space (quiet time to yourself to allow for introspection)

One of the most powerful tools yet greatest distractions we all have today is our cell phone. Be aware of how its use is helping or hindering your mindfulness journey. This ten-day period might be the ideal time to step away from social media or practice putting your phone away for one hour before bed—you be the judge!

If you're like us and you have small children or a bustling environment, remember that meditation and mindfulness are not about striving for serene silence for easy focus. It's about finding calm amid the chaos! The more difficult and challenging it is for you, the more you just need to focus on practice (not perfection)!

REST	READ AND WRITE	RECONNECT	REFLECT
DAY 21	devotional + journal—three things you're grateful for	reconnect—10-min. meditation	reflect—what was your energy level like today?
DAY 22	devotional + journal—a favorite childhood memory	reconnect—go barefoot outside	reflect—what emotion(s) did you primarily experience today?
DAY 23	devotional + journal—where do you see yourself in five years?	reconnect—call a friend to catch up	reflect—did you feel mindful and intentional today?
DAY 24	devotional + journal—a favorite quote and what it means to you	reconnect—turn on a favorite song and dance	reflect—what worked well today? Successes?
DAY 25	devotional + journal—a difficulty you've overcome	reconnect—do five min. of breath work	reflect—what can you do better tomorrow?
DAY 26	devotional + journal—what gets you most excited?	reconnect—choose one fruit or veggie and practice mindful eating	reflect—do you feel like you live more in the past or future? How can you be more present?
Day 27	devotional + journal—ten compliments to yourself	reconnect—write a special note to a friend online	reflect—what made you feel tense today? What made you feel relaxed?
Day 28	devotional + journal—three most impactful moments in your life	reconnect—notice all five senses and which is strongest	reflect—what inspired you today?

| Day 29 | devotional + journal— what your perfect day would look like | reconnect—do a full-body stretch for 5 min. | reflect—what time of day are you most productive? Do you enjoy most? |
| DAY 30 | devotional + journal— someone or something you're inspired by and why | reconnect—go for a 10-min. walk outside | reflect—how does time outside make you feel? |

Eat Move Rest: Days 31 to 40

The last and final ten days will be all yours! Continue to eat plant-based meals and make room for daily exercise and mindfulness. Follow our suggested meal, movement, and mindfulness plans or adapt them to make them work better for you. The difference here is all in your mindset. At this point, you should be feeling more independent, confident, and empowered and experiencing some of the benefits highlighted earlier on.

Rather than looking forward to crossing the finish line, this is your time to figure out how to make these new habits a *lifestyle* that you can sustain. Reflect on what's been working and what hasn't. Give it your all in this final stretch, and when you're done, journal about your experience.

Day 41 (and Beyond)!

Congratulations—you did it! This isn't the end, it's just the beginning! We hope you're feeling amazing! It's time to look in the mirror and give yourself a pat on the back for completing not just a diet challenge but a total lifestyle shift. This is something you can own for life if you choose to. Continue to nurture your mind, body, and soul on a consistent basis and let the results be your motivation. The way you feel should be enough to keep the momentum going. And when you fall down, get back up and just keep moving forward, no matter the pace. You did it, and you can keep doing it, better and better each and every day!

Love how you feel? We want to hear from you—connect with us on social media and share your experience!

Keep it going! Join our Eat Move Rest Club, which includes all our ebooks, helpful handouts, access to the Eat Move Rest meal planner and recipe app, inclusion in our private Facebook group, live chats, coaching, and connection! Learn more at EatMoveRest.com.

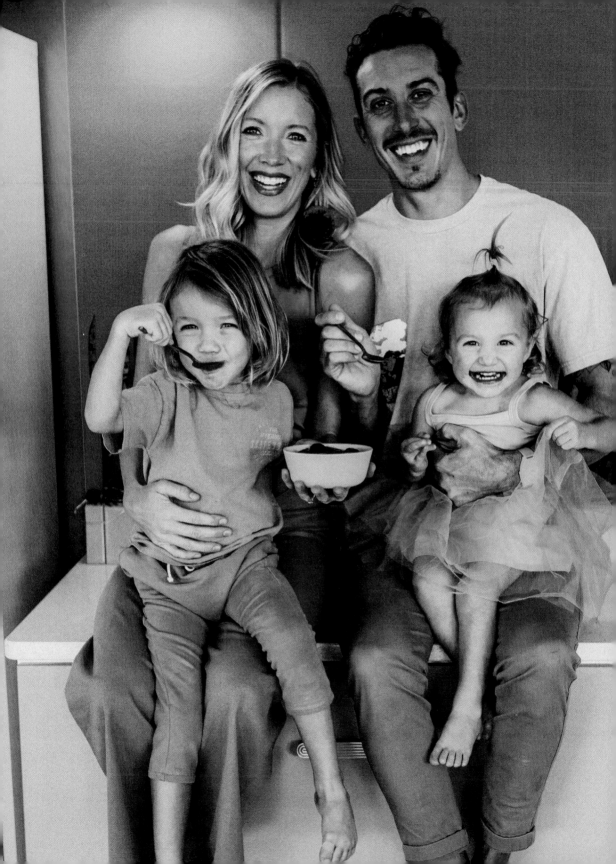

Part Three
The Recipes

Now that we've shared our Eat Move Rest philosophy *and* the brass tacks of how to stay afloat on a plant-based diet, it's time to dive in! Coming up are our absolute favorite-tasting and most-nutrient-dense recipes and meals that we feel will deliver maximum benefit to you. We place a heavy emphasis on incorporating lots of elevating, colorful, raw living foods into our days and grounding, hearty cooked foods into our evenings. Get ready to have some flavorful fun as you juice, blend, and chop your way into an abundantly nourished life!

All recipes are oil-free and refined sugar–free and will have a gluten-free and soy-free option.

Use the following key to help you find the right recipe for you:

(K) = Kid-friendly favorites

Note: Because the overwhelming majority of our recipes are "kid friendly" (with the exception of the Ginger Turmeric Cure-All Shot!), we decided that the K label on certain recipes would indicate our kids' *absolute* faves in each recipe category.

(R) = Raw / no cooking

(DIY) = Make it your own. The training wheels are off!

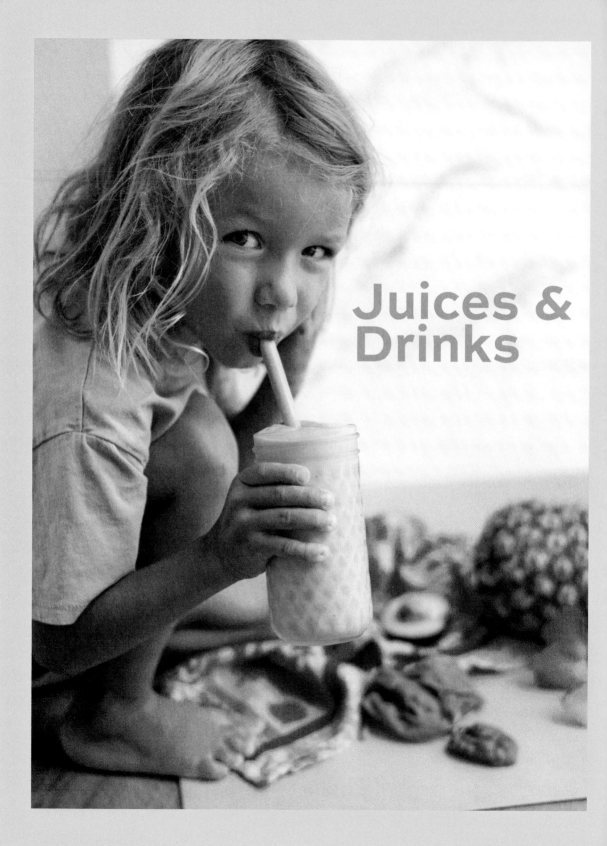

Juices & Drinks

We like to view juicing through a medicinal lens and each delicious drink in this section serves a powerful purpose. While we typically want fiber to remain intact, juicing is the exception. When the hydrating, nutrient-dense liquid is extracted from the pulp, you're left with a highly concentrated dose of vitamins, minerals, antioxidants, and enzymes. When the digestive system is able to rest from processing all that "bulk," those nutrients are better able to quickly and easily enter into the bloodstream and cells where they can go to work healing, repairing, and energizing.

ALL RECIPES ARE (R).

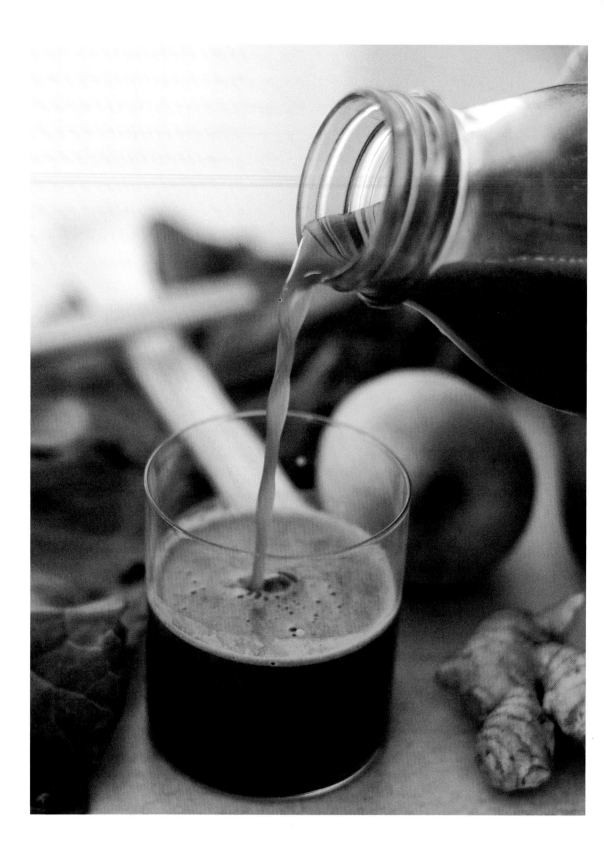

Green Machine Detox Juice

We make this juice recipe more than any other. It's an epic alkalizing elixir if you've overindulged or if you just feel like you need a salad in a glass! The key to making this juice extra juicy is adding more cucumber and celery, as they are the most water-dense ingredients and will increase the volume quickly.

(R) | SERVES 2 | TIME: 15 MINUTES

1- to 2-inch piece fresh ginger, unpeeled
½-inch slice fresh turmeric, unpeeled
Handful fresh parsley
1 head romaine lettuce leaves
5 or 6 large leaves lacinato (dinosaur) kale
2 or 3 unpeeled cucumbers, chopped

1 head celery, with the root end trimmed
1 lemon, peeled
1 fennel bulb (optional, but great for additional digestive support)
1 Granny Smith apple, cored and chopped (optional, for a touch of sweetness)

In a juicer, place the ginger, turmeric, parsley, romaine leaves, kale, cucumbers, celery, and lemon as well as the fennel and apple (if using). Enjoy the juice right away or refrigerate in an airtight container for up to 48 hours.

Note: For an extra-smooth juice, pour through a fine-mesh strainer to eliminate any excess pulp. You can also juice the ginger and turmeric separately and drink as a shot! (See Ginger Turmeric Cure-All Shot page 71.)

Sweet Green Energy Juice

This is the ideal green juice to get your gut used to greens, especially if you can't stomach the taste! The pineapple and green apple totally eliminate any hint of bitterness and adding fruit provides a little extra oomph of energy.

(R) | SERVES 2 | TIME: 15 MINUTES

5 or 6 large leaves lacinato (dinosaur) kale
3 or 4 large leaves collard greens
Handful fresh cilantro (optional)
2 or 3 unpeeled cucumbers, sliced

1 head celery, with the root end trimmed
1 lemon, peeled
1 or 2 Granny Smith apples, cored and chopped
1 to 2 cups chopped fresh pineapple

In a juicer, place the kale, collard greens, cilantro (if using), cucumbers, celery, lemon, apple, and pineapple. Sip the juice right away or refrigerate in an airtight container for up to 48 hours.

Note: For an extra-smooth juice, pour through a fine-mesh strainer to eliminate any excess pulp.

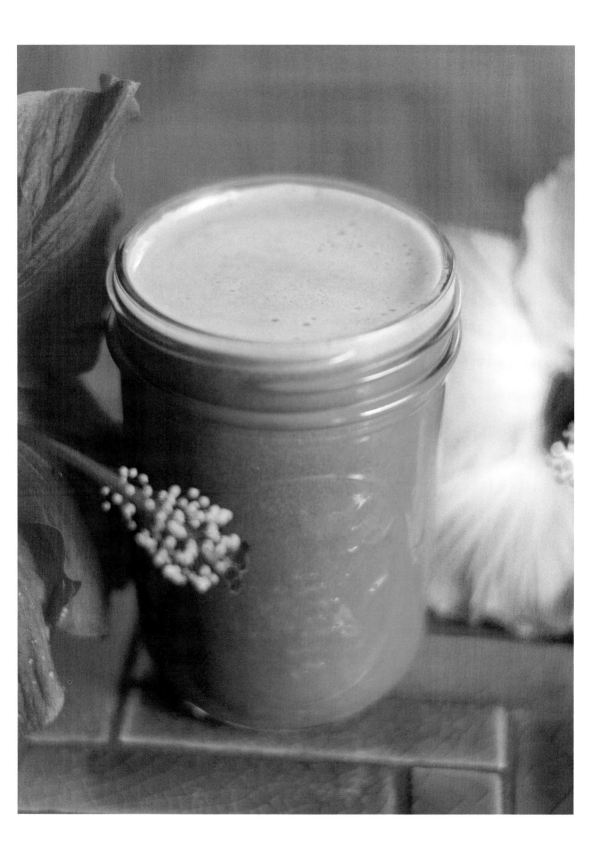

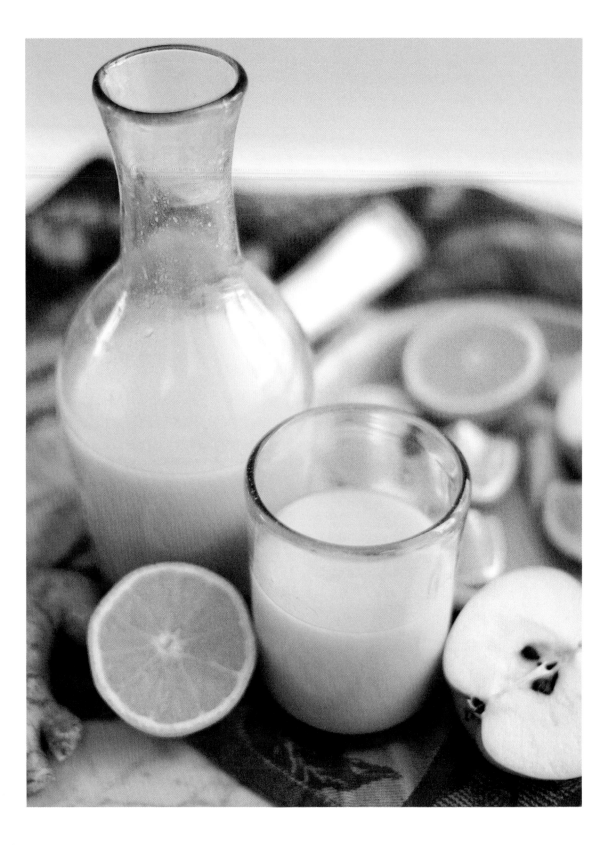

Liquid Gold Immunity Juice

This sunshine in a glass is high in vitamins A and C and is fantastic for optimal digestion, glowing skin, and boosting the immune system. It also boasts a bounty of anti-inflammatory benefits. This one is a powerhouse!

(R) | SERVES 2 | TIME: 15 MINUTES

5 oranges, peeled

2 to 3 cups chopped fresh pineapple

1- to 2-inch piece fresh ginger, unpeeled

½-inch slice fresh turmeric, unpeeled

2 Granny Smith apples, cored and chopped

2 stalks celery

In a juicer, place the oranges, pineapple, ginger, turmeric, apples, and celery. Drink right away or refrigerate the juice in an airtight container for up to 48 hours.

> **Note:** For an extra-smooth juice, pour through a fine-mesh strainer to eliminate any excess pulp.

ABC Active Juice

ABC—Apple Beet Carrot—juice is ideal before a long run or an epic lift session. Beets help to oxygenate your blood, and the sweet natural sugars will amp up your sweat sesh. Add a bit of ginger to lower inflammation and really get your guns fired up!

(R) | SERVES 1 TO 2 | TIME: 10 MINUTES

1 or 2 medium Granny Smith apples, cored and chopped

2 or 3 (3-inch) beets, unpeeled

3 carrots, unpeeled

½-inch piece fresh ginger, unpeeled (optional)

In a juicer, place the apples, beets, carrots, and ginger (if using). Drink the juice right away or refrigerate in an airtight container for up to 48 hours.

> **Note:** For an extra-smooth juice, pour through a fine-mesh strainer to eliminate any excess pulp.

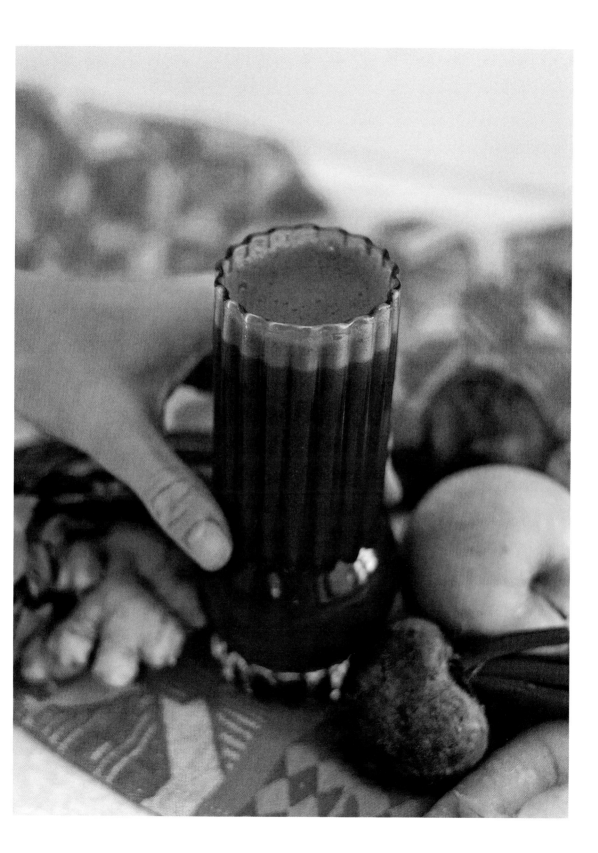

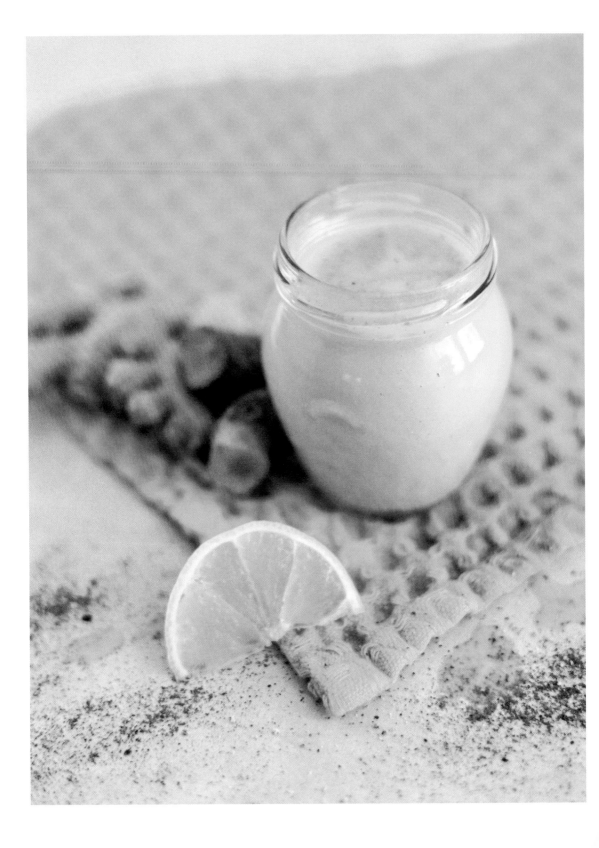

Ginger Turmeric Cure-All Shot

This simple shot can help to reduce inflammation, chronic pain, and nausea, as well as support immune function. Plus, it clears the sinuses and gives you an instant jolt of energy! Sip this first thing in the morning after a late night or at the hint of a sniffle or sore throat. Need a chaser to wash down this shot? A lemon or orange slice will do the trick.

(R) | SERVES 2 | TIME: 5 MINUTES

¼ cup chopped fresh ginger, unpeeled
¼ cup chopped fresh turmeric, unpeeled
1 lemon, peeled

Crack of freshly ground black pepper
Dash of cayenne pepper
Slice of lemon or orange

1. In a juicer, place the ginger, turmeric, and lemon.
2. Top the juice with black pepper and cayenne and gulp down right away.
3. Chase with a slice of lemon or orange. Store any extra ginger, turmeric, and lemon juice in an airtight container for up to 48 hours.

Note: For an extra-smooth juice, pour through a fine-mesh strainer to eliminate any excess pulp.

Mermaid Lemonade

Sometimes your water just needs a little something to make it fun to drink, and this bright, hydrating, detoxifying, and tasty combo does the trick. Spirulina is extremely nutrient-rich, and you'll recognize just how potent it is the moment you mix up your drink and see the beautiful color it imparts! A pinch of sea salt will also help to restore trace minerals and electrolytes on hot summer days.

(R) | SERVES 1 | TIME: 3 MINUTES

12 ounces fresh filtered water
⅛ teaspoon blue spirulina powder
Juice of 1 lemon, plus additional
thin lemon slices, for serving

1 teaspoon maple syrup (optional)
Pinch of sea salt
Ice cubes, for serving

1. In a glass, add the water, spirulina, lemon juice, maple syrup (if using), and salt and mix well.
2. Pour the mixture into another glass filled with ice and sip this refreshing and hydrating beverage with additional thin lemon slices for garnish. Keeps well in the refrigerator in an airtight container for up to 48 hours.

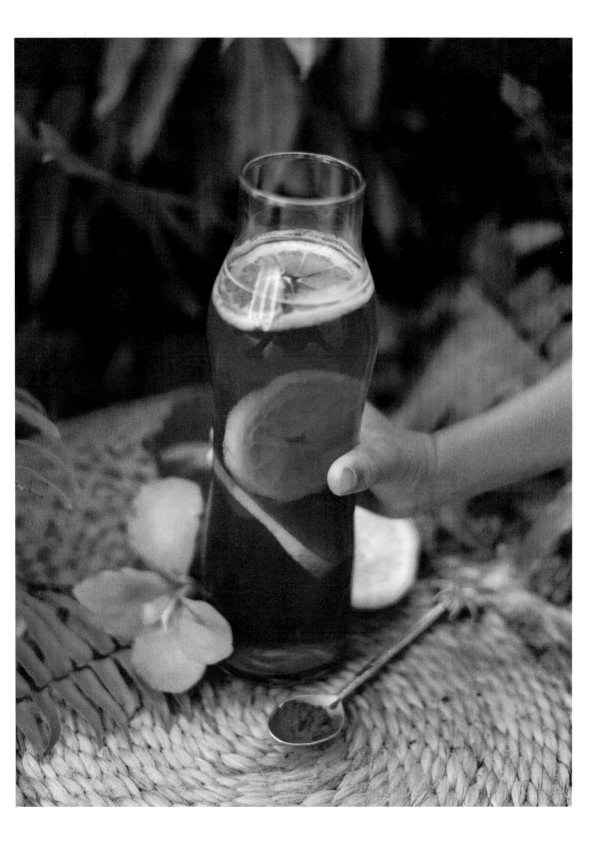

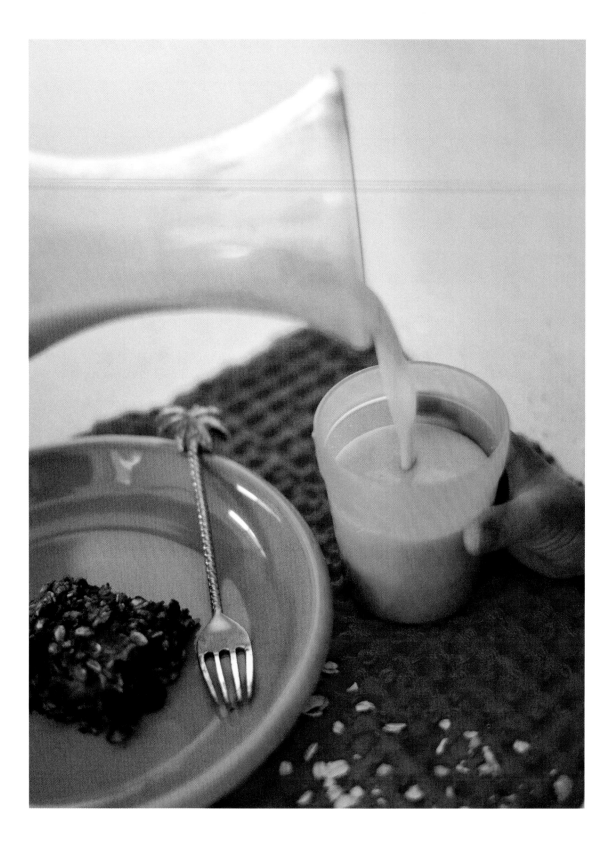

Creamy Vanilla Plant Milk

This simple recipe is free of any preservatives and other unwanted ingredients that many store-bought plant milks contain. Many raw nuts and seeds work well, and oats are another favorite. We recommend trying almonds, cashews, hemp seeds, or rolled oats. This beverage is best enjoyed alongside our Baked Berry Oats recipe (page 108).

(R) (DIY) | SERVES 6 | TIME: 6 TO 8 HOURS (FOR SOAKING NUTS AND SEEDS) + 10 MINUTES

1 cup raw nuts, seeds, or rolled oats (see Note)
2 to 3½ cups filtered water, plus more for soaking
1 teaspoon vanilla bean powder or
½ to 1 teaspoon vanilla extract

Pinch of pink sea salt
3 to 6 Medjool dates, pitted and soaked for at least 20 minutes in warm water
¼ teaspoon ground cinnamon

1. Soak the nuts or seeds in filtered water overnight (6 to 8 hours) and then drain and rinse. If you are using rolled oats, soaking is not necessary.
2. Place the nuts, seeds, or oats into a high-speed blender, add 2 cups of the filtered water as well as the vanilla, salt, dates, and cinnamon, and blend until smooth. Add more water as needed to achieve the desired consistency.
3. Into a large bowl, strain the liquid through a nut milk bag or cheesecloth. Squeeze out as much excess liquid as possible. Pour a glass of the milk alongside your favorite oat dish and store extra in an airtight container in the refrigerator for 4 to 5 days.

Note: Even though oats are naturally gluten-free, they are often contaminated with gluten-containing ingredients during processing. To be sure your oats are free of gluten, look for a gluten-free label.

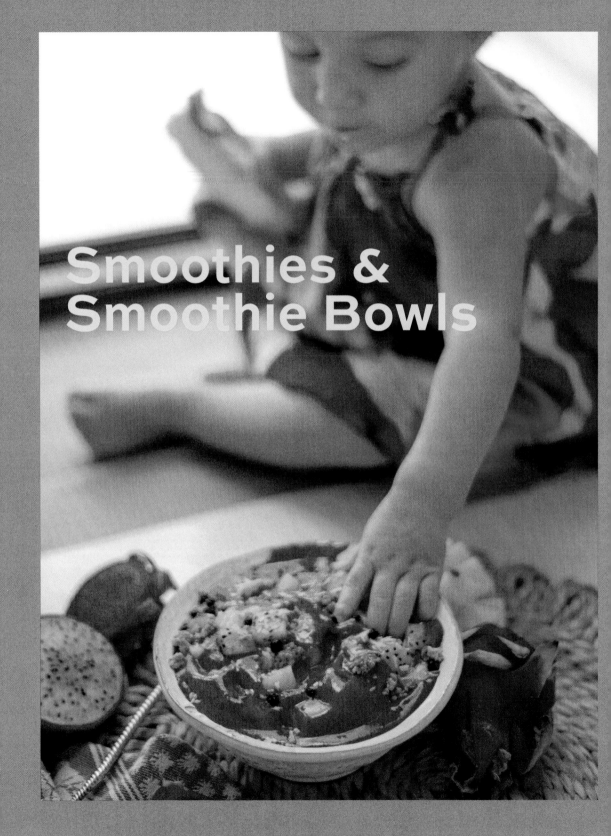

Smoothies &
Smoothie Bowls

We consider smoothies and smoothie bowls a daily staple. They're quick, easy, nutrient-dense, and delicious. When we were having trouble developing a taste for kale, blueberries, and other plant foods rich in phytonutrients, we began hiding them in smoothies and over time, the gut adapted! Every blend in this section tastes like a dessert that you can enjoy any time of day. Either sip these smoothies through a straw on-the-go or blend them a bit thicker and enjoy by the spoonful topped with your favorite superfoods!

ALL RECIPES ARE (R).

Go Bananas!

Call us monkeys, but bananas are a definite staple around here. . . . So much so that we buy them by the case. A case contains about ninety to one hundred bananas, and this will last us two to three weeks as a family of four. Not only will you receive a discount from most grocery stores for buying in bulk, but they also keep remarkably well in the freezer. Bananas form the base of (nearly) every creamy and sweet smoothie we make!

If you have a sensitivity, intolerance, or simply can't get on board with naners, try replacing them with frozen mango instead. A lower calorie replacement option would be cauliflower.

If you're not a fan, before you give up on bananas, make sure you're enjoying them when they are actually ripe. (Most smoothie shops use unripe bananas that disappoint, taste- and texture-wise.)

Ripe means a speckled, freckled, and leopard-spotted peel—not to the totally brown peel and super mushy "banana bread point" but a couple of days before then. If there is any green, they are not ready, and more time is needed to allow the starches to convert into sugars. This is going to make your smoothies taste less "banana-y" and more sweetly satisfying.

Frozen Banana Prep

1. Allow the bananas to ripen.

2. Peel them.

3. Break each banana into three or four pieces.

4. Place the bananas on a parchment-lined baking sheet or in a reusable plastic bag or container and pop into the freezer.

5. To use in a smoothie, remove the bananas from the freezer and, if they are sticking together, use a spoon to break them apart (we keep one in the freezer for easy access).

6. When blending frozen bananas with other ingredients, we find it most effective to add them last and opt to add ingredients that are easier to blend toward the bottom, closest to the blade (see the How to Build a Smoothie infographic on the opposite page). This allows the blender to blend more efficiently without the motor burning out or the blades becoming dull.

how to:
build a smoothie

From the bottom up, here's how to build a perfect plant-powered smoothie that'll blend with ease!

6 Fresh or Frozen Fruit
Ripe bananas, apple, pineapple, mango, papaya, kiwi, peach, berries, cherries, citrus, pitaya

5 Leafy Greens & Veggies
Spinach, kale, romaine, chard, collards, cucumber, celery, beets, carrots, cauliflower

4 Healthy Fats
Hemp, chia, flax, sesame, avocado, nuts, coconut milk and cream, nut butter

3 Quality Protein
Plant-based (vegan) protein powder (hemp, brown rice, pea, soy)

2 Superfoods
Ginger, turmeric, moringa, maca, spirulina, matcha, camu, cacao, açaí, wheatgrass, barley grass, dates

1 Liquid
Water, coconut water, fruit juice (orange, apple), plant milk (almond, coconut)

Try our Go-To Green Protein Smoothie (page 81) for an epic combo!

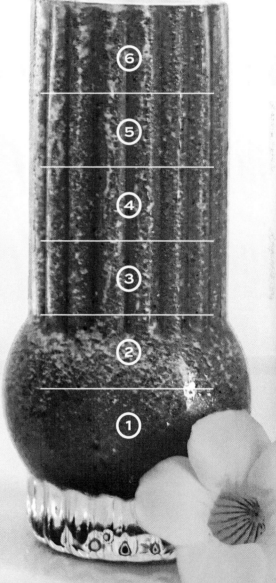

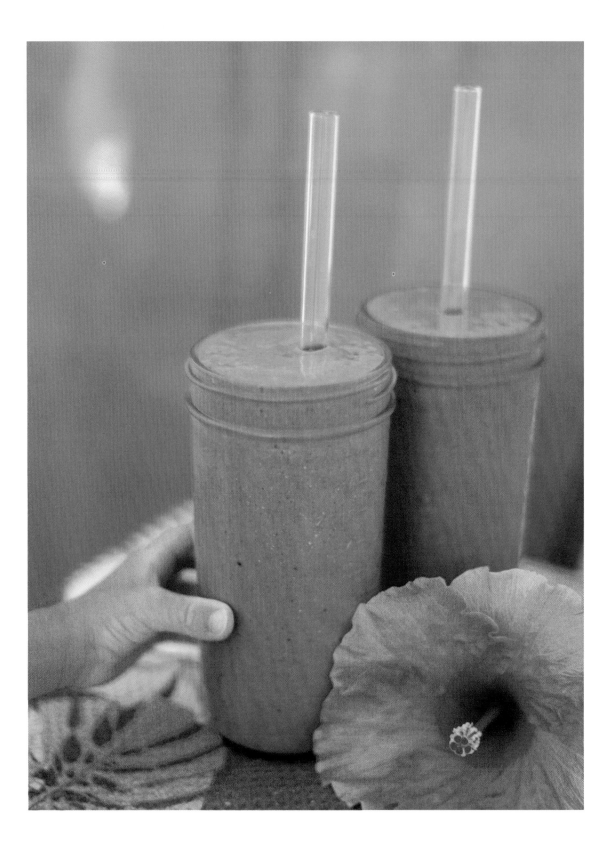

Go-To Green Protein Smoothie

We love smoothies because they're easy to grab and go. This is our absolute favorite green smoothie recipe of all time, and we drink it almost every morning! Even the kiddos love this one, and it's a sneaky way to get more greens into their gut. It tastes amazing while providing a wide variety of essential nutrients including omega-3s (flax and chia), iron (dulse, barley grass–juice powder, spirulina), selenium (Brazil nut), iodine (dulse), protein, and lots more. It's a multivitamin (and a salad) in a glass!

(R) | SERVES 2 | TIME: 10 MINUTES

3 cups filtered water

1 raw Brazil nut

1 thin coin-size slice fresh ginger, unpeeled

1 thin coin-size slice fresh turmeric, unpeeled, or dash of ground turmeric (optional)

2 tablespoons whole flaxseeds or chia seeds

½ tablespoon dulse flakes

1 heaping tablespoon barley grass–juice powder or spirulina

1 scoop vanilla plant-based protein powder (optional)

5 or 6 large leaves lacinato (dinosaur) kale

2 celery stalks

1½ cups frozen or fresh pineapple chunks

1 to 2 cups frozen mango chunks

1 Granny Smith apple, cored and chopped

3 frozen ripe bananas

Place the water, Brazil nut, ginger, turmeric (if using), flaxseeds, dulse flakes, barley powder, protein powder (if using), kale, celery, pineapple, mango, apple, and bananas in a high-speed blender and blend until smooth. This smoothie is best consumed immediately but can be refrigerated in an airtight container for 24 hours or frozen for several days.

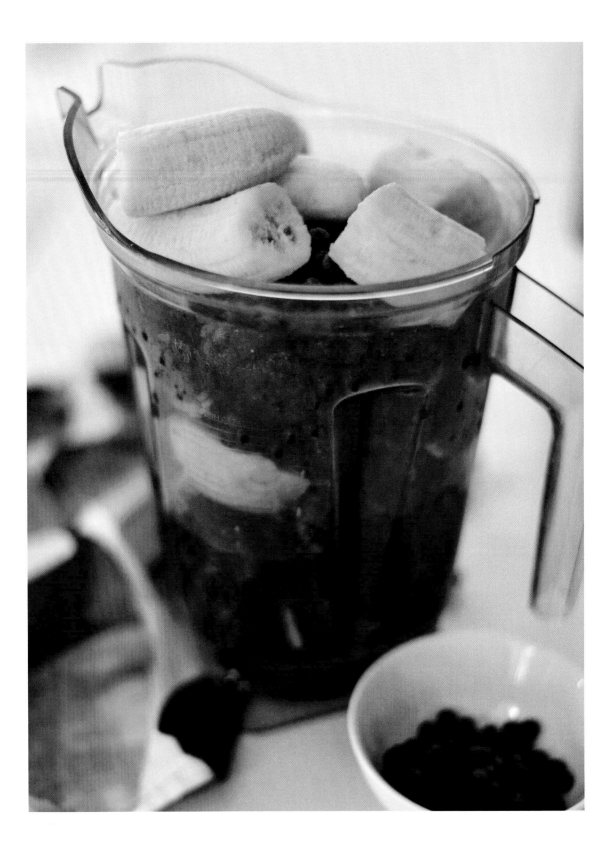

Wild Blueberry Detox Green Smoothie

This smoothie tastes incredible, and it will work some magic! Wild blueberries are much higher in antioxidants than regular blueberries, and spirulina is highly detoxifying and mineral-rich. Most mornings we alternate between this smoothie and our Go-To Green Protein Smoothie (page 81).

(R) | SERVES 2 | TIME: 10 MINUTES

2½ cups filtered water
2 tablespoons chia seeds or flaxseeds
1 tablespoon dulse flakes
1 tablespoon spirulina
2 dashes of ground cinnamon
1 scoop chocolate plant-based protein powder (optional)

2 celery stalks
2 handfuls spinach leaves
2 cups frozen wild blueberries
3 frozen ripe bananas

Place the water, chia seeds, dulse flakes, spirulina, cinnamon, protein powder (if using), celery, spinach, blueberries, and bananas in a high-speed blender and blend until smooth. The smoothie is best consumed immediately but can be refrigerated in an airtight container for 24 hours or frozen for several days.

How to Boost Your Blends

PROTEIN

- Amp up any smoothie or smoothie bowl with a high-quality plant-based protein powder. Visit our faves page at EatMoveRest.com/Our-Faves to see our recommendations.
- Alternatively, add a whole food protein like hemp seeds or silken tofu.

ENHANCERS

- For more sweetness add: vanilla or chocolate plant-based protein powder, freshly squeezed orange juice, coconut water, or pitted, soaked Medjool dates.
- For extra creaminess and thickness add: avocado, coconut milk or cream, or hemp seeds.
- For tartness add: lemon, lime, or passion fruit.

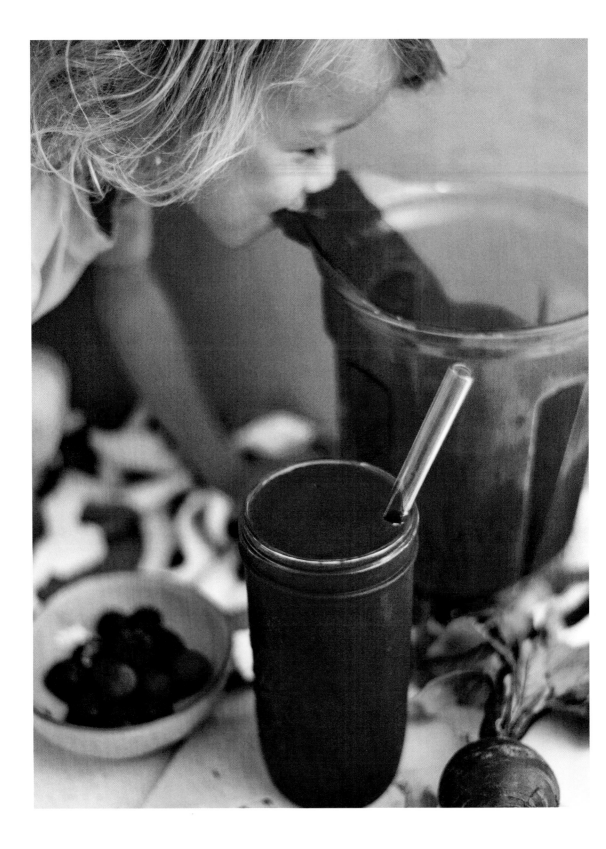

Un-Beetable Preworkout Smoothie

This blend is the best sip for getting sweaty. Beets are known to oxygenate the blood, thanks to their nitrates. This equates to running farther, jumping higher, and overall performing better for longer. Cherries are a rich source of antioxidants and maca is adaptogenic. This total package will help to fuel you preworkout and heal you postworkout.

(R) | SERVES 2 | TIME: 10 MINUTES

2 cups coconut water

2 teaspoons maca powder

2 tablespoons hemp seeds

1 scoop chocolate plant-based protein powder (optional)

1 medium beet, unpeeled, with beet greens

2 cups frozen cherries

3 frozen ripe bananas

Place the coconut water, maca, hemp seeds, protein powder (if using), beet and beet greens, cherries, and bananas in a high-speed blender and blend until smooth. This smoothie is best consumed immediately but can be refrigerated in an airtight container for 24 hours or frozen for several days.

Note: If omitting the protein powder, consider adding ½ tablespoon cacao powder for chocolate flavor.

Tangerine Dream Immunity Smoothie

This blend is like sunshine in a glass! It's loaded with immunity-boosting vitamins A and C, and it'll help to combat sniffles, sore throats, and coughs. Thanks to anti-inflammatory ginger and turmeric, this smoothie is also effective at recovering from any aches or pains.

(R) | SERVES 2 | TIME: 10 MINUTES

2 tangerines or 1 cup orange juice

1 scoop vanilla plant-based protein powder (optional)

1 cup frozen or fresh pineapple chunks

1 large carrot, unpeeled

1 thin coin-size slice fresh ginger, unpeeled

1 thin coin-size slice fresh turmeric or ½ teaspoon ground turmeric

1 cup frozen mango

2 frozen ripe bananas

3 tablespoons coconut cream (optional)

Place the tangerines, protein powder (if using), pineapple, carrot, ginger, turmeric, mango, bananas, and coconut cream (if using) in a high-speed blender and blend until smooth. This smoothie is best consumed immediately but can be refrigerated in an airtight container for 24 hours or frozen for several days.

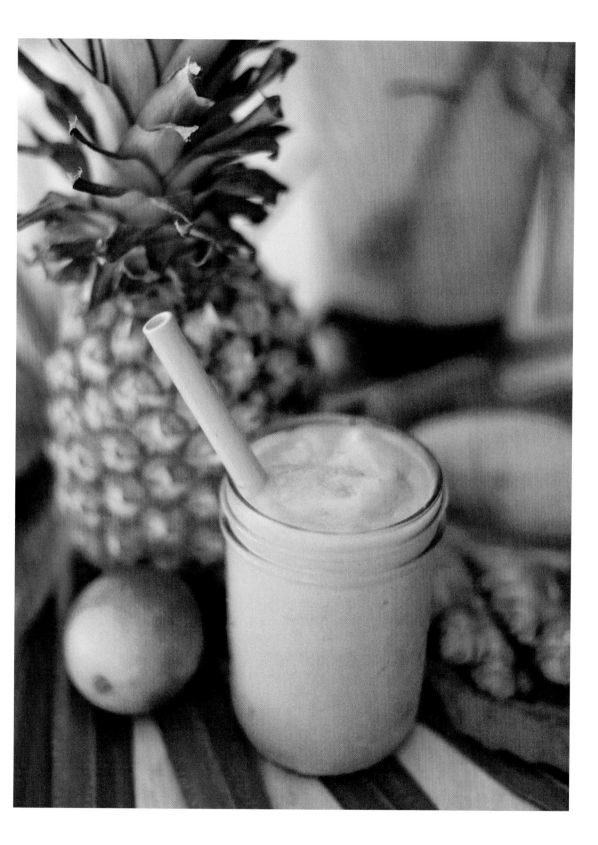

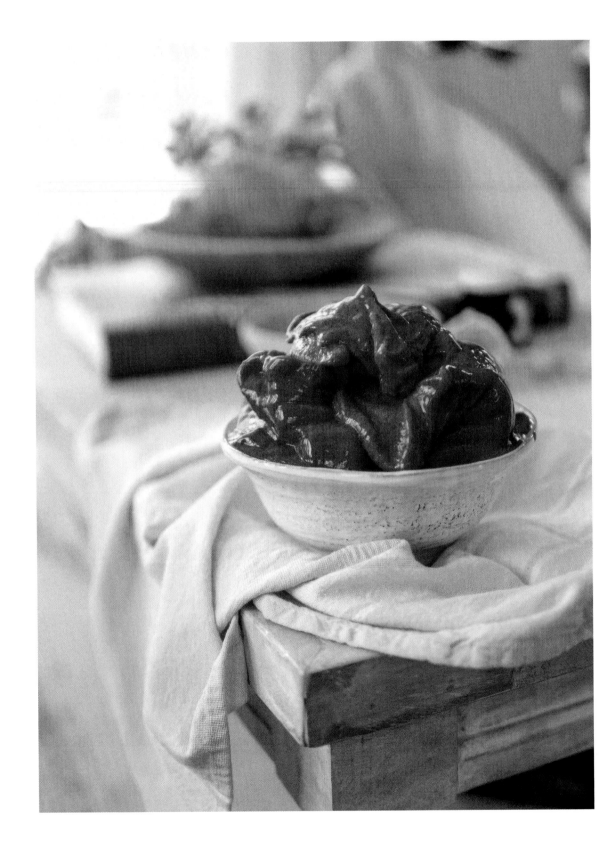

Pink Bubble Gum
Smoothie Bowl

Sometimes blends are better slurped by the spoonful rather than sipped through a straw. Smoothie bowls and nice creams offer a thicker and creamier consistency and make for an enjoyable sit-down meal topped with all your favorite fruits and superfoods. You won't believe this blend until you try it! This smoothie bowl tastes just like bubble gum thanks to jackfruit. Legend has it, jackfruit gave Juicy Fruit bubble gum its original flavor.

(R) (K) | SERVES 2 | TIME: 10 MINUTES

1 scoop vanilla plant-based protein powder (optional)

1 cup frozen raspberries

1 cup frozen strawberries

4 frozen ripe bananas

1 cup frozen mango

7 frozen jackfruit pods

1 frozen pitaya (dragon fruit) pack or a small chunk of beet, unpeeled, for color

1 to 2 cups filtered water

Place the protein powder (if using), raspberries, strawberries, bananas, mango, jackfruit, pitaya, and water in a high-speed blender and blend until smooth. Start with a minimal amount of liquid, adding more as needed, until blended to a thick, creamy consistency. This smoothie bowl is best consumed immediately but can be refrigerated in an airtight container for 24 hours or frozen for several days.

Note: It can be helpful to allow the frozen ingredients to thaw for 5 to 10 minutes before blending so your blender doesn't overheat and to make blending easier.

Build Your Own Açaí or Pitaya Smoothie Bowl

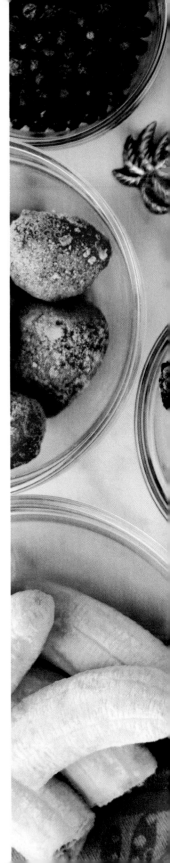

If you're looking for a sweet, Instagram-able treat, an açaí or pitaya smoothie bowl is your best bet! These brightly hued antioxidant-rich ingredients will do wonders for your skin and your immune system and will help to combat the damage to cells caused by free radicals. The best part is a bowl made with either of these powerhouses and sprinkled with the toppings of your choice tastes like a dessert with benefits!

(R) (DIY) | SERVES 2 | TIME: 10 MINUTES

1 cup coconut water

1 scoop vanilla or chocolate plant-based protein powder (optional)

2 cups frozen berries of choice

1 frozen açaí or pitaya pack or 1 tablespoon açaí or pitaya powder

4 frozen ripe bananas

Fresh or dried fruit, nuts, seeds, and superfoods of choice, for topping (see Note below)

1. Place the coconut water, protein powder (if using), berries, açaí, and bananas in a high-speed blender and blend until smooth.
2. Pour the smoothie into a bowl, add your desired toppings, and dig in. The smoothie bowl is best consumed immediately but can be refrigerated in an airtight container for 24 hours or frozen for several days.

Note: Toppings we love include hemp seeds, cacao nibs, shredded coconut, freeze-dried strawberries, dried mulberries, and dried goji berries.

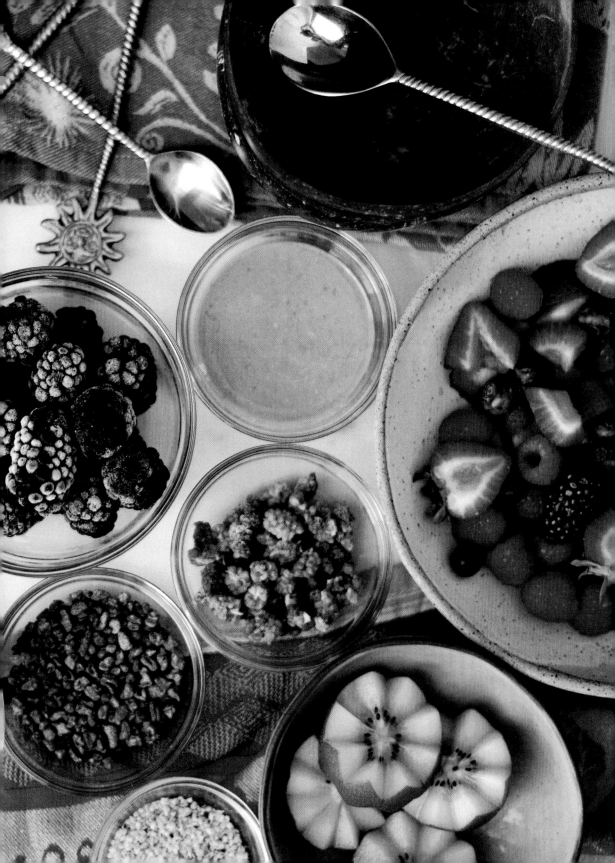

Peanut Butter Date Smoothie Bowl

This dairy-free delight tastes just like a candy bar, but you can eat it for dessert or for breakfast—it's *that* healthy!

(R) | SERVES 2 TO 3 | TIME: 5 MINUTES

Splash of plant milk

6 frozen ripe bananas

4 Medjool dates, pitted and soaked for at least 20 minutes in warm water

2 tablespoons cacao powder

2 tablespoons peanut butter or peanut butter powder

1 scoop chocolate plant-based protein powder (optional)

Sweet cacao nibs, hemp seeds, sliced Medjool dates, and a drizzle of peanut butter, for topping (optional, for extra deliciousness!)

Place the plant milk, bananas, dates, cacao powder, peanut butter, and protein powder (if using) in a high-speed blender and blend until smooth and creamy. Add your desired toppings. The smoothie bowl is best consumed immediately but can be refrigerated in an airtight container for 24 hours or frozen for several days.

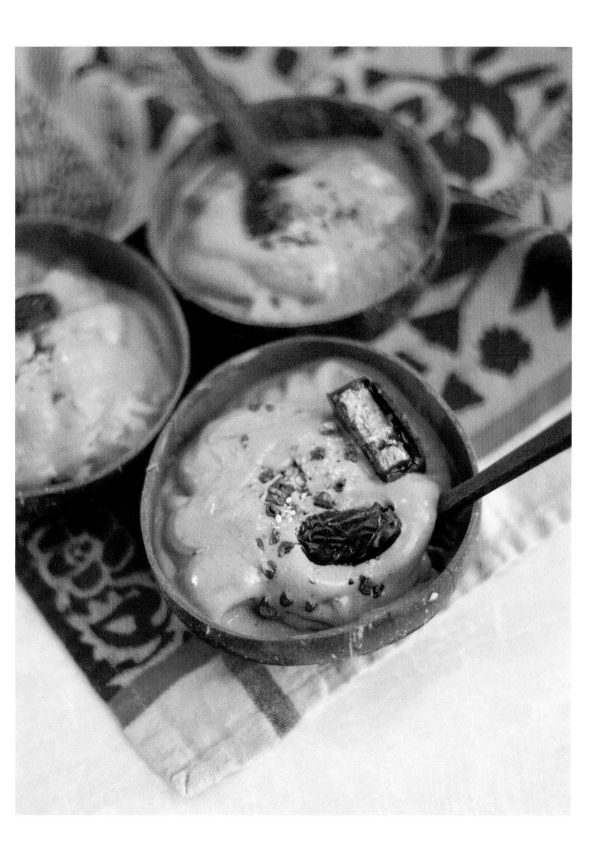

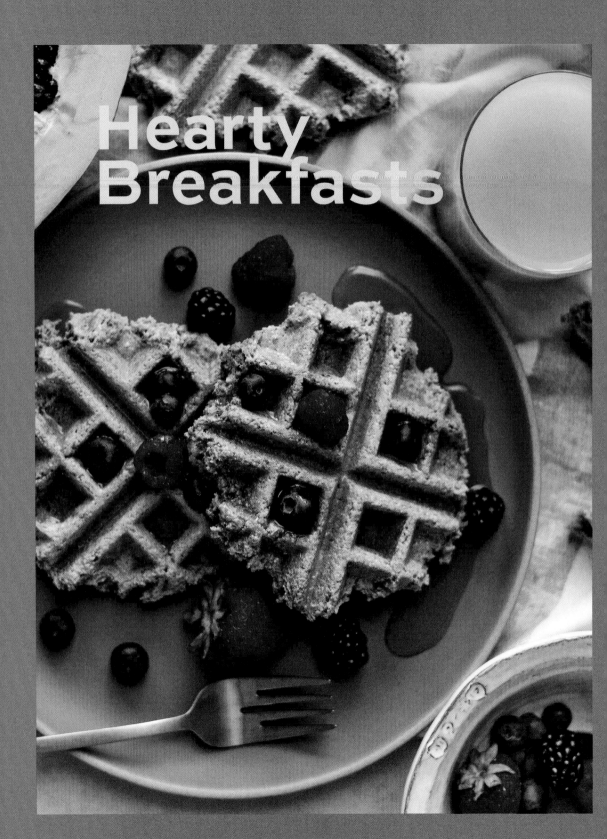

Hearty
Breakfasts

We live by the saying "Eat breakfast like a king, lunch like a queen, and dinner like a pauper." That means we fill up for breakfast to fuel our day. The perfect counterpart to a refreshing juice or smoothie is a hearty breakfast bowl like our Chocolate Cherry Rolled Oats (page 99) or our Veggie-ful Breakfast Scramble (page 100). Oats are so versatile, we use them often in many different creative ways to keep it fun and interesting (especially for our little ones), and there are plenty of oat-free options, as well!

Fantastic Fruit Plate

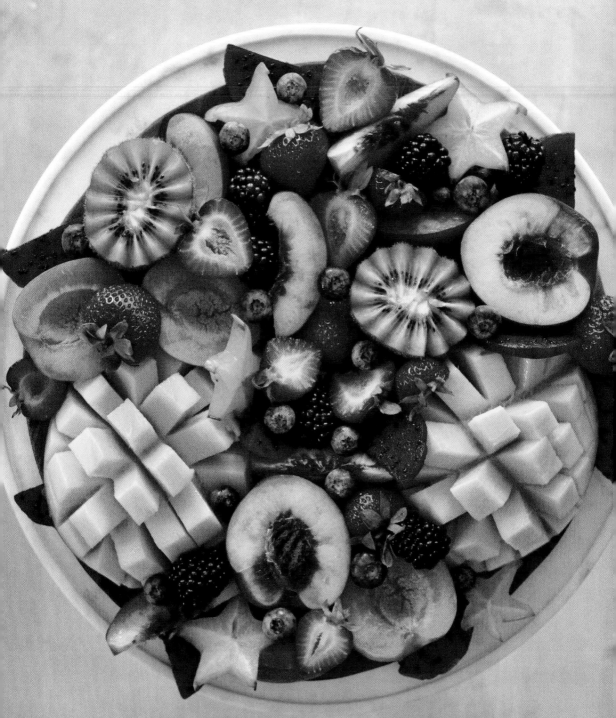

The simplest form of carbohydrate energy—otherwise known to us as nature's candy, a natural "fruit snack," weapons of mass nutrition, fast fruit, and brain food—is *fruit*!

The nice thing about eating fruit is that you can eat as much as you desire, and your body will let you know when it is satiated without leaving you feeling like you overdid it. If you would like to recalibrate your mind and body to recognize what true hunger and true satiety feel like, try a mono-meal. Pick just one ripe, seasonal fruit and eat as much of it as you want. When your body says stop, you're done!

These are the most important things to keep in mind when it comes to eating and enjoying fruit:

- Shop for seasonal (most important!), organic (when possible), and local (if possible).
- Buy ripe fruit, or allow fruit to ripen at home before eating. Here's a quick ripeness guide to some of our favorite fruits:
  - Bananas are ripe when there are leopard spots on the skin.
  - Mangoes are ripe when slightly soft to the touch.
  - Pineapples are ripe when fragrant and/or the skin is yellow.
  - Oranges are best when the skin is soft but not pulling away from the inside.
  - Watermelon is best when you can see a yellow spot on one side.

For optimal digestion, fruit is always best consumed by itself. Including fats and proteins can slow the process. Smoothies are an exception. Even though they usually contain a mix of fruits, fats, and proteins, they are easy to digest because the food has been broken down and is essentially one step digested (prechewed) already.

(R) (DIY) | SERVES AS MANY AS YOU WANT! | TIME: 10 TO 20 MINUTES, DEPENDING ON NUMBER AND TYPES OF FRUITS USED

Berries	Bananas	Watermelon	Peaches
Cherries	Pineapple	Cantaloupe	Nectarines
Kiwi	Oranges	Mangoes	Star fruit

Arrange artfully on a plate or board. Let your creativity run free!

Save Your Skins!

Did you know you can eat the skins, tops, and cores of many fruits? We love to eat kiwis with the skin on—with a good rinse and scrub, they're good to go! Strawberry tops are another one. Have you ever noticed that after you slice the tops off, the discard pile is as big as the eat pile? And the core of the pineapple is the highest source of bromelain, which is highly anti-inflammatory. A great way to make use of these "scraps" is to pop them in the freezer and add them to your next smoothie for added nutrition and to get more bang for your buck!

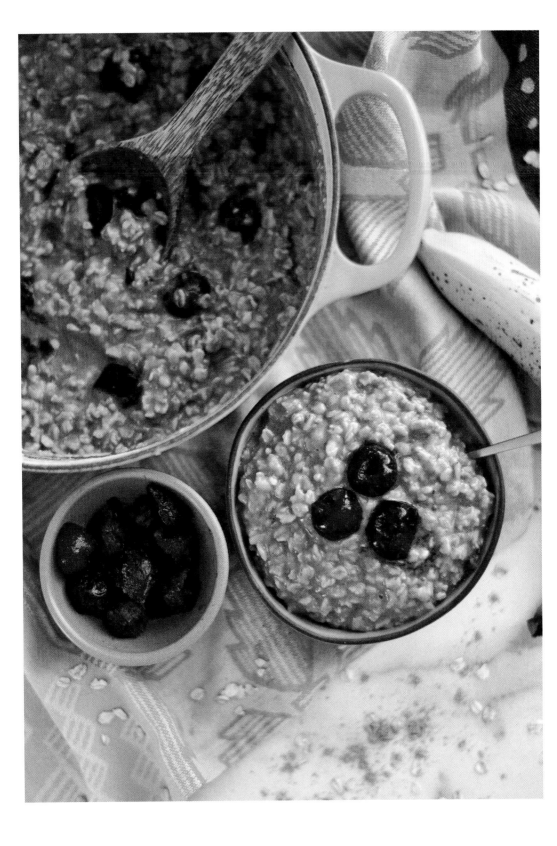

Chocolate Cherry Rolled Oats

Oats are a staple almost every morning in our household, but when we don't have time for pancakes, waffles, or steel-cut or baked oats, this is our quickest fix. The chocolate-cherry combo has been a fan favorite around here for quite some time, and warm oats are the perfect counterbalance to a nice chilled fruit smoothie!

SERVES 4 | TIME: 10 MINUTES

2 cups filtered water
2 cups plant milk
2 cups rolled oats
½ teaspoon ground cinnamon
Pinch of sea salt

2 fresh ripe bananas, mashed
1 cup frozen cherries
1 scoop chocolate plant-based protein powder or 1 tablespoon cacao powder and 1 tablespoon maple syrup or 4 pitted Medjool dates, chopped

1. To a large pot, add the water, plant milk, oats, cinnamon, and salt and bring to a boil. Reduce the heat to medium-low and simmer, stirring often, for 7 minutes or until fluffy and thick.
2. Add the bananas, cherries, and protein powder and stir to combine. Enjoy with a glass of Creamy Vanilla Plant Milk (page 75) or your favorite juice recipe. The oats keep best in an airtight container in the refrigerator for up to 3 days.

Veggie-ful Breakfast Scramble

This high-protein, cholesterol-free upgrade is sure to please anyone! On-the-go? Scoop your scramble up and fold it into a wrap! If you're looking for a soy-free alternative that's also high in protein, try using a can of chickpeas in place of tofu.

SERVES 2 TO 3 | TIME: 10 MINUTES

½ yellow sweet onion, diced

2 garlic cloves, minced

1 (14-ounce) block extra-firm tofu or 1 (15.5-ounce) can chickpeas, drained and rinsed

½ red, orange, or yellow bell pepper, diced

Handful cherry tomatoes, diced

1½ tablespoons nutritional yeast

¼ teaspoon ground turmeric

Sea salt and freshly ground black pepper to taste

Handful spinach leaves, chopped

2 or 3 slices Ezekiel 4:9 sprouted whole grain bread, toasted, for serving

1. Add a splash of filtered water to a large frying pan over high heat and sauté the onion and garlic until both are translucent.
2. Add the tofu, using a fork to smash the block into smaller chunks and crumbles. If you are using chickpeas, add them to the pan and mash with a fork.
3. Add the bell pepper, cherry tomatoes, nutritional yeast, turmeric, salt, and pepper and stir to combine.
4. Cook for 10 minutes, stirring occasionally.
5. Remove from the heat, add the spinach, and mix until the spinach turns dark green. Plate with a side of sprouted Ezekiel 4:9 toast. Store leftovers in an airtight container in the refrigerator for up to 3 days.

Note: Add 1 cup cooked quinoa and/or ½ cup black beans to the scramble to boost the nutrition even more!

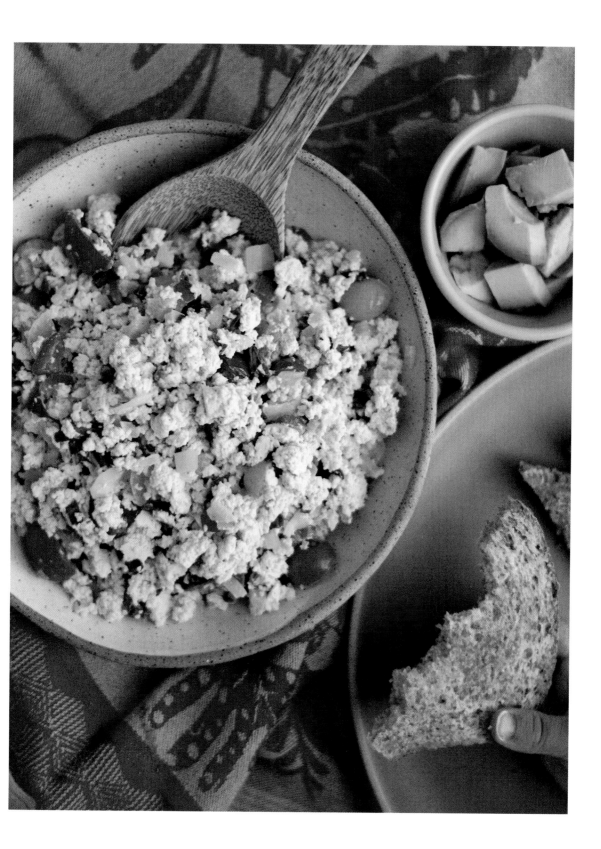

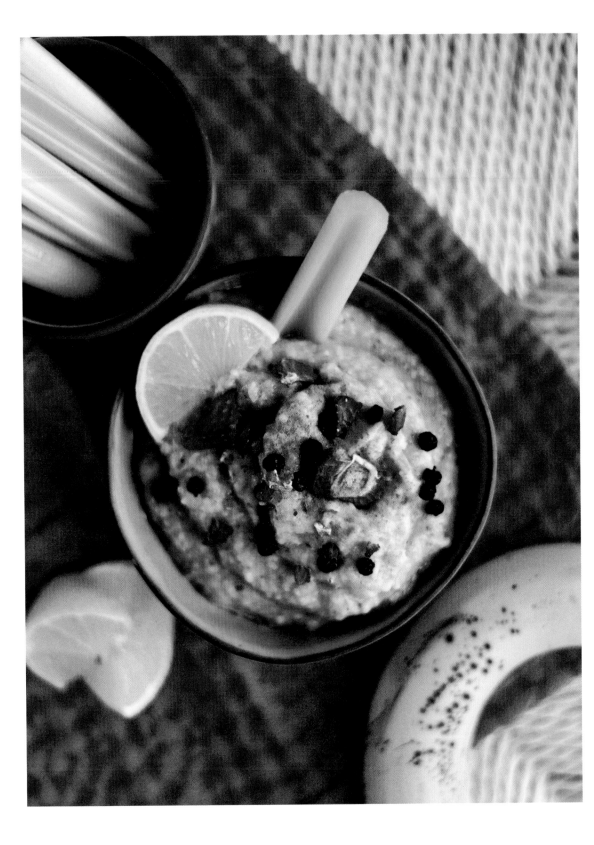

Apple Banana Date Porridge

This is a favorite breakfast, snack, or anytime meal that looks just like its cooked counterpart, but it's totally raw! Think of it as extra-fancy applesauce.

(R) | SERVES 1 | TIME: 5 MINUTES

1 unpeeled Honeycrisp apple, cored and chopped

1 fresh ripe banana, chopped

2 or 3 Medjool dates, pitted and soaked for at least 20 minutes in warm water

Juice of ½ lemon

Fresh or dried fruit, raw nuts, seeds, and superfoods of choice, for topping (see Note below)

Celery sticks, for serving (optional)

1. Add the apple, banana, dates, and lemon juice to a food processor and pulse until the mixture is the consistency of oatmeal or porridge.
2. Pour the mixture into a small bowl and enjoy with a sprinkle of your favorite toppings. Try using celery sticks to scoop, crunch, and enjoy—seems odd, but trust us, it's deeelish! This porridge is best enjoyed immediately.

Note: We like to top this porridge with hemp seeds, freeze-dried strawberries, and dried blueberries.

Banana Oat Waffles

This maple-infused breakfast classic is one of our kiddos' favorites. L'Eggo your Eggo and try this simple fix instead. Add a handful of berries or a generous spread of cashew butter and a drizzle of maple syrup on top for the Max special!

(K) | SERVES 4 TO 5 | TIME: 10 MINUTES

2 cups rolled oats

2 tablespoons chia seeds

2 teaspoons vanilla bean powder or 1 scoop vanilla plant-based protein powder

2 teaspoons baking powder

Pinch of sea salt

2 fresh ripe bananas

2 tablespoons maple syrup

1 cup plant milk

Coconut oil or vegan butter, for the waffle iron

Maple syrup and fresh berries, for topping

Freshly squeezed orange juice, for serving

1. Place the rolled oats and chia seeds in a high-speed blender and blend until smooth. Add to a large mixing bowl along with vanilla protein powder or vanilla bean powder, baking powder, and salt and set aside.
2. Place bananas, maple syrup, and plant milk in high-speed blender and blend until smooth. Add to large mixing bowl along with dry ingredients and stir to combine.
3. Preheat the waffle iron, coat it with a thin layer of oil or vegan butter to prevent sticking, and pour in batter. Cook for 2 to 3 minutes, or until golden and crisp. Repeat this process until all the batter has been cooked.
4. Plate and serve with a drizzle of maple syrup, a sprinkle of berries, and a side of freshly squeezed orange juice. Leftovers keep best in an airtight container in the refrigerator for up to 3 days.

Note: We use a ceramic coated waffle iron that does not require the use of oil or vegan butter and it works like a charm!

Also Note: This recipe can be used to make pancakes.

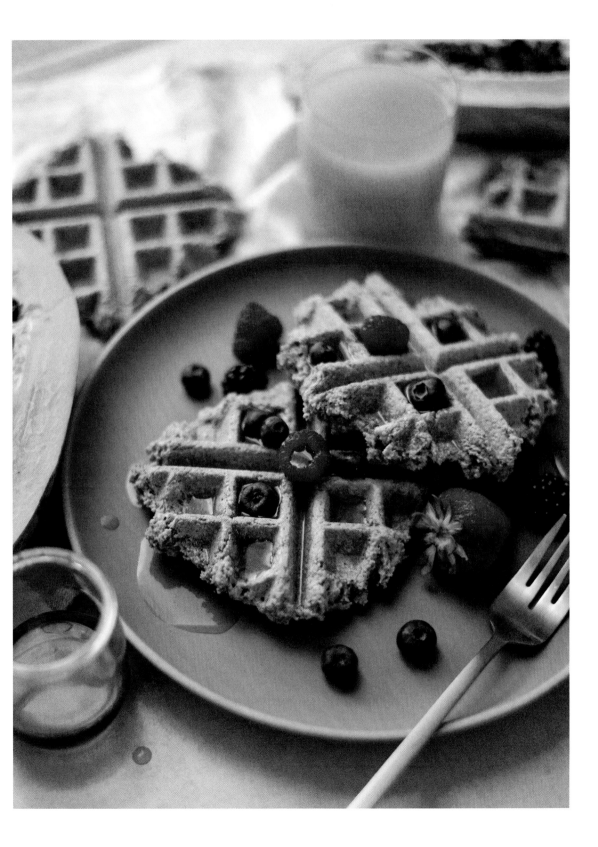

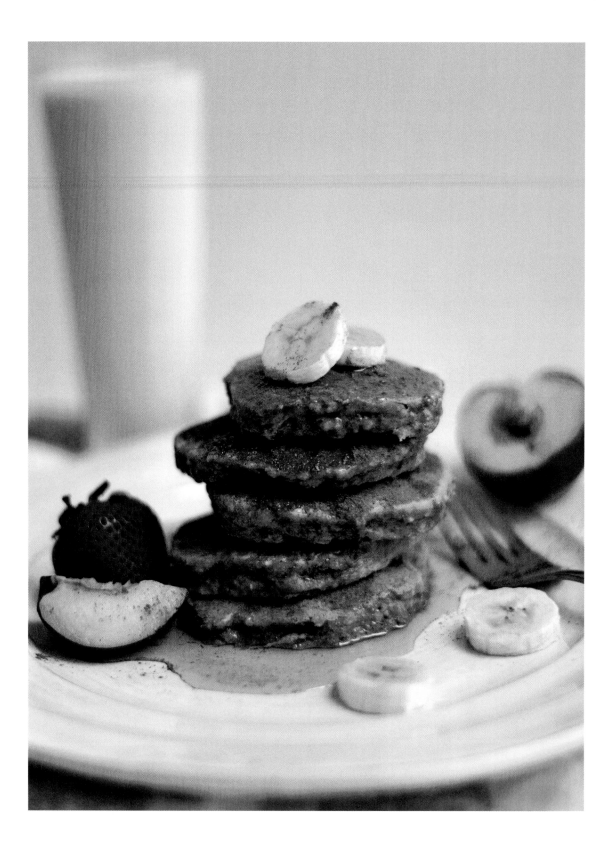

Flip-Free Protein Pancakes

Buckwheat is a nutritious alternative to try in place of oats for baking. It's a complete protein that's also rich in iron. Sprinkle in some additional plant-based protein powder and these pancakes really become a flippin' powerhouse! But wait, did we mention these can actually be made no-fuss and flip-free?!

SERVES 6 TO 8 | TIME: 10 MINUTES

2 cups buckwheat groats
2 tablespoons chia seeds and/or flaxseeds
1 scoop vanilla plant-based protein powder or 2 teaspoons vanilla bean powder
2 teaspoons baking powder
Pinch of sea salt

1½ cups plant milk
2 fresh ripe bananas
2 tablespoons maple syrup, plus more for topping
Fresh fruit, for topping
Creamy Vanilla Plant Milk (page 75), for serving

1. Preheat the oven to 350°F. Line a baking sheet with parchment paper.
2. Place the buckwheat groats and seeds into a high-speed blender and blend until a fine flour is achieved. Add the mixture to a large mixing bowl along with the protein powder, baking powder, and salt. Mix well and set aside.
3. Place the plant milk, bananas, and maple syrup in a high-speed blender and blend until smooth. Add the plant-milk mixture to the bowl with the dry ingredients and mix until well combined.
4. Pour ¼ cup portions of the batter onto the prepared baking sheet to form rounds. Bake for about 15 minutes or until the pancakes are slightly golden on top and cooked in the middle. Remove from the oven and allow to cool on the baking sheet for 5 minutes.
5. Plate with fresh fruit, such as strawberries, bananas, and nectarines and a drizzle of maple syrup, and serve with a side of Creamy Vanilla Plant Milk. Store leftovers in an airtight container in the refrigerator for up to 3 days.

> **Stovetop Alternative:** Heat a large nonstick pan over medium heat. Pour ¼ cup portions of the batter into the pan. Flip after cooking for about 1 minute, or when bubbles begin to form and pop. Cook the second side for 1 to 2 minutes, or when the underside is golden brown, and transfer to a plate.
>
> If sticking occurs between batches, take a paper towel and "wax on, wax off" a thin layer of coconut oil. This small amount of oil is less about dietary consumption and more about achieving the ideal end product!

Baked Oats Two Ways

If you're bored with your everyday stovetop oatmeal, try this baked version! Enjoy the crispy, golden top and creamy center, hot out of the oven, or allow the oats to cool and firm up into a barlike consistency for a finger-licking good snack. Whether you're in the mood for berry or banana bread flavor, both versions are rich in protein, antioxidants, and healthy omega-3 fatty acids and taste like dessert for breakfast!

SERVES 15 | TIME: 40 MINUTES

2 fresh ripe bananas
2 tablespoons chia seeds
2 cups rolled oats
2 tablespoons maple syrup, plus more for topping
2 cups oat milk

2 teaspoons baking powder
Dash of sea salt
2 teaspoons ground cinnamon
2 tablespoons cashew butter, plus more for topping

Baked Berry Oats

1 to 2 cups frozen mixed berries
2 teaspoons ground cinnamon

Banana Bread Baked Oats

4 to 6 pitted Medjool dates, chopped
1 teaspoon pumpkin pie spice

Additional fresh slices of banana, for topping

1. Preheat the oven to 375°F.
2. Add the bananas and chia seeds to a high-speed blender and blend until smooth.
3. Transfer the mixture to a large mixing bowl and add the rolled oats, maple syrup, oat milk, baking powder, salt, cinnamon, and cashew butter. If you are making the Baked Berry Oats, also add the frozen mixed berries and additional cinnamon. If you are making the Banana Bread Baked Oats, add instead the dates and pumpkin pie spice. Mix until well combined.
4. Transfer the oat mixture to a baking dish (and top with sliced bananas for Banana Bread Baked Oats). Bake for 30 minutes or until the top is golden brown. Remove from the oven and let cool for 5 to 10 minutes.
5. Serve right away for a runnier consistency or let the oats cool longer and slice into bars. The kiddos especially enjoy this dish topped with a drizzle of maple syrup and a dollop of cashew butter. The baked oats keep well in an airtight container in the refrigerator for up to 3 days.

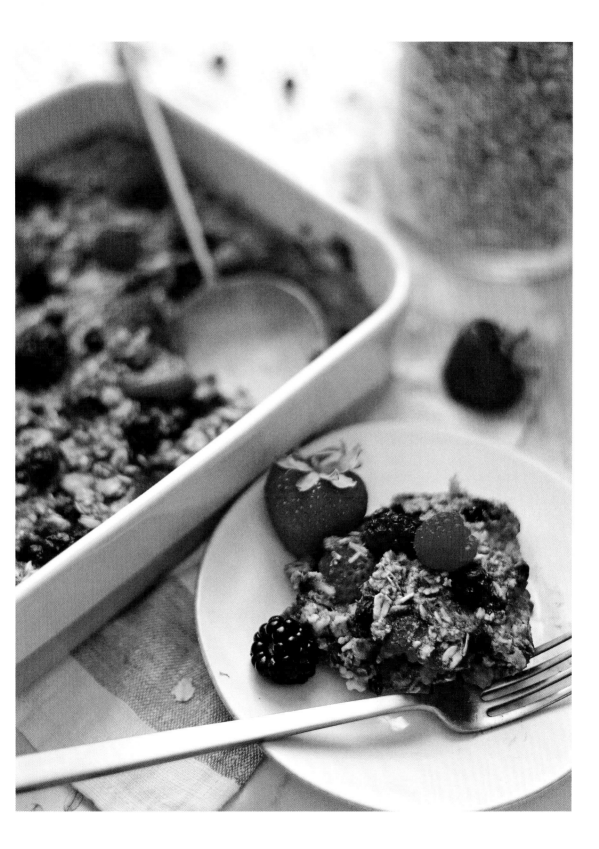

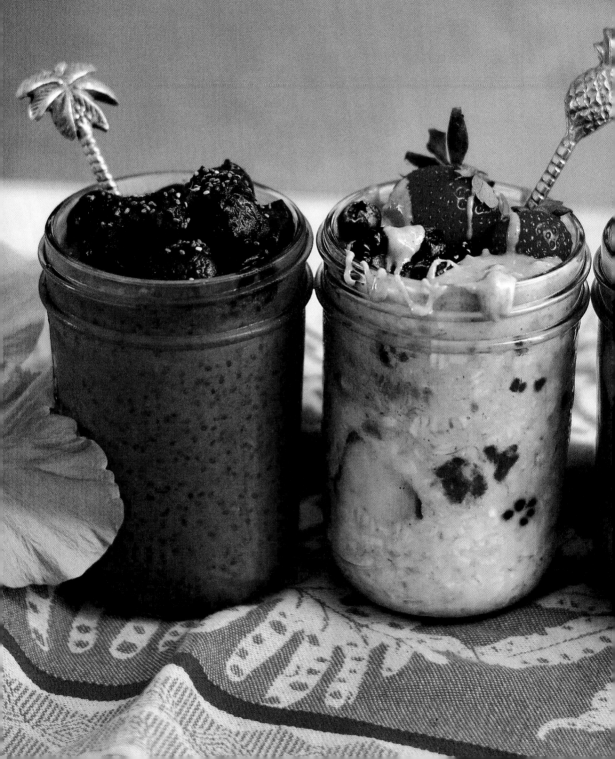

On-the-Go Duo

Overnight oats and chia pudding are two of our favorite meals to whip up on the fly because they take minutes to make ahead of time and keep well in mason jars in the refrigerator. Both are concentrated sources of nutrition and calories, meaning they'll keep you fueled up wherever your day takes you. Make them in advance and store in the refrigerator for up to 3 days.

Chocolate Chia Seed Pudding

This fluffy, omega-3-rich meal-in-a-jar boasts a uniquely satisfying texture and is super energizing, thanks to chia.

(R) | SERVES 1 | TIME: 30 MINUTES

1 fresh ripe banana

2 teaspoons cacao powder

1 cup plant milk (we like oat or soy)

Pinch of sea salt

2 pitted Medjool dates or 1 tablespoon maple syrup (optional, for added sweetness)

½ scoop chocolate plant-based protein powder (optional)

¼ cup chia seeds

Small handful frozen or fresh cherries, for topping

1. Place the banana, cacao powder, plant milk, salt, dates, and protein powder (if using) in a high-speed blender and blend until smooth.
2. Pour the mixture into a wide-mouthed mason jar and mix in the chia seeds. Secure the lid and pop in the refrigerator for at least 3 hours or up to overnight. Top with fresh or frozen cherries and enjoy!

Vanilla Bean Overnight Oats

If you're a vanilla person, this creamy, dreamy recipe is for you. Take this recipe to the next level with a dollop of nut butter and a handful of berries. It'll taste just like the PB&J of your childhood!

(R) | SERVES 1 | TIME: 5 MINUTES

1 fresh ripe banana, mashed

1 cup plant milk (we like oat or soy)

½ teaspoon vanilla bean powder or vanilla extract

½ scoop vanilla plant-based protein powder (optional)

Pinch of sea salt

¾ cup rolled oats

½ cup fresh or frozen berries

2 Medjool dates, pitted and chopped, or 1 tablespoon maple syrup (optional, for added sweetness)

Nut butter, fresh berries, homemade granola, hemp seeds, or chia seeds, for topping (optional)

1. In a large bowl, mix the banana, plant milk, vanilla, protein powder (if using), and salt.
2. In a wide-mouthed mason jar, place the milk blend, rolled oats, berries, and dates (if using). Mix thoroughly. Cover and place in the refrigerator for at least 3 hours or up to overnight.
3. Drizzle with nut butter and add a sprinkle of berries or your choice of toppings.

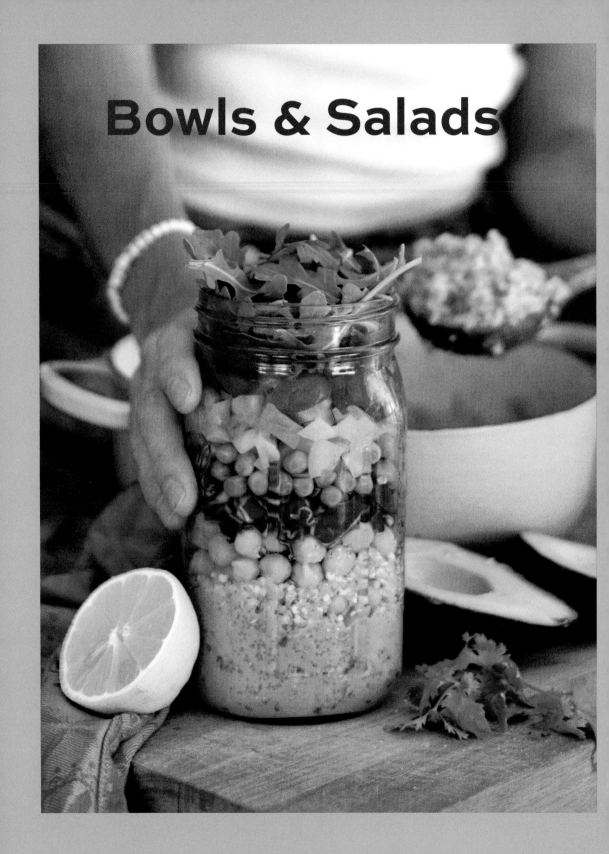

Bowls & Salads

We love incorporating as much color into our meals as possible, and our bowls and salads showcase this perfectly. Not only are the colors of the rainbow beautiful and appetizing, they also unlock a full spectrum of nutrients in each and every juicy, crunchy bite. You can expect plenty of flavor in this section and a healthy combination of raw and cooked plant foods that are ideal for lunch or dinner.

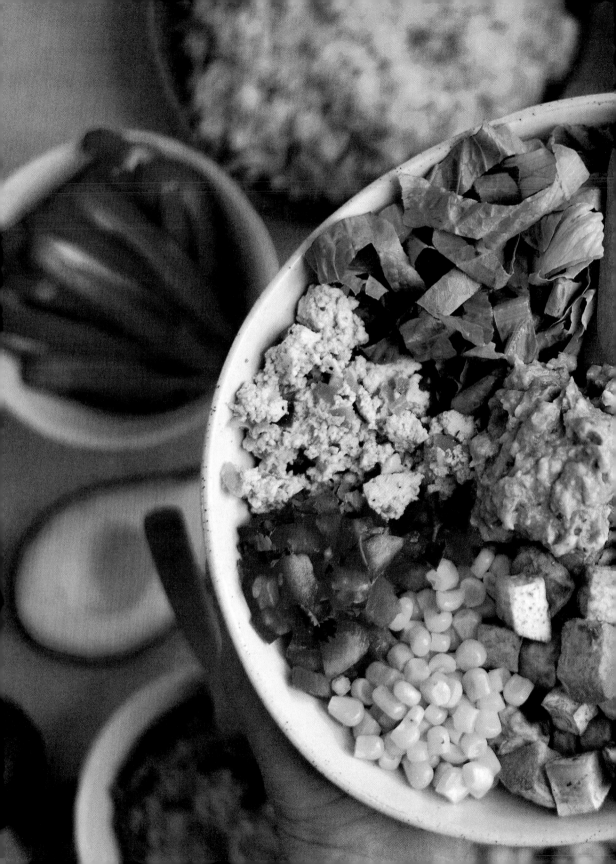

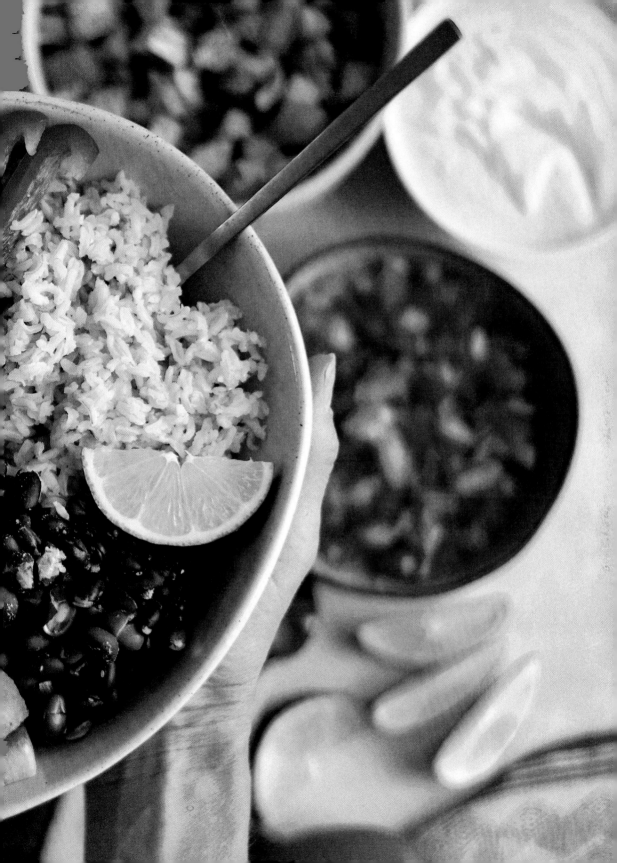

Better-for-You Burrito Balance Bowl

This is hands down our family's favorite balance bowl. Even though there are a lot of components, they're all easy and effortlessly thrown together. Many of them can be prepped ahead of time and kept in containers in the refrigerator, so that they are ready to combine for a quick and nourishing lunch or dinner. So many flavors, so much nutrition!

SERVES 4 TO 6 | TIME: 45 MIN

3 medium sweet potatoes, cut into 1-inch cubes

Sea salt and freshly ground black pepper to taste

1 (14-ounce) block extra-firm tofu (or try our Red Lentil Tofu, page 117)

Taco sauce or hot sauce to taste (we like Red Duck or Yellowbird)

1 red onion, chopped

3 garlic cloves, chopped

1 head romaine lettuce, shredded

3 cups cooked brown rice

3 cups cooked black beans (see page 118)

1 bell pepper, chopped

1 cup sweet corn kernels

1 batch Grateful Green Guacamole (page 215)

1 batch Creamy Cashew Cheeze (page 219)

1 batch Perfect Pico de Gallo (page 218)

Fresh cilantro leaves and lime wedges, for garnish

Large tortillas, for serving (optional)

1. Preheat the oven to 400°F. Line a baking sheet with parchment paper.
2. Add the sweet potatoes to the prepared baking sheet and season with salt and pepper. Spread the potatoes in an even layer and bake for 25 to 30 minutes, until the potatoes are fork-tender, tossing halfway through.
3. Add a splash of water to a large sauté pan over medium heat and add the extra-firm tofu. Mash the tofu with a fork until it resembles a scramble, and season with salt, pepper, and taco sauce.
4. Add a splash of water to a medium frying pan over medium heat and sauté the onion and garlic until softened.
5. To build your bowls, divide the lettuce leaves, sweet potatoes, tofu (sofritas), onion, garlic, rice, beans, bell pepper, sweet corn, guacamole, cashew cheeze, and pico de gallo between bowls. Garnish with cilantro and lime and serve! Or divide the ingredients among large tortillas and roll into a burrito for a handheld version. Leftovers keep best in individual airtight containers for up to 3 days.

*Soy-Free Option: Red Lentil Tofu

We are firm believers in the benefits of organic soy, as it has been shown to have protective properties against two of the most common forms of cancer, breast and prostate. However, if your preference is to opt for soy-free alternatives, or you're looking for a homemade alternative to store-bought tofu, this protein and iron-rich Red Lentil Tofu recipe is a tasty protein to add to a balance bowl and is sure to become a household staple!

SERVES 4 | TIME: 48 HOURS (FOR SOAKING LENTILS AND SETTING MIXTURE) + 30 MINUTES

+ 30 MINUTES

1 cup red lentils
2 cups boiling filtered water
½ tablespoon sea salt

2 cups room-temperature filtered water (see Note below)
Coconut aminos (optional)

1. In a large bowl, cover the lentils with water and soak overnight.
2. Drain and rinse the lentils and place them back in the large bowl. Add the boiling water and allow the lentils to soak for 20 minutes.
3. Add the lentils-water mixture and salt to a high-speed blender and blend until smooth.
4. Pour the blended lentils into a large pot and whisk in the room-temperature water. Bring the lentils to a boil over medium-high heat. Reduce the heat to medium-low and simmer for about 10 minutes while whisking continuously until a thick, creamy consistency is achieved. The mixture will begin to clump onto the whisk.
5. Remove from the heat and pour into a large baking dish. Allow to cool at room temperature and then cover and place in the refrigerator overnight.
6. Cut into cubes and eat as is or season with coconut aminos and bake in the oven at 400°F for 15 minutes, tossing halfway through. Remove from the oven and allow to cool for 5 minutes. Enjoy by itself or add to your favorite savory dish. Keeps well in an airtight container in the refrigerator for up to 5 days.

Note: This recipe will make a firm tofu. For an extra-firm tofu, add only 1 cup room-temperature water.

Beans, Beans

We prefer to cook our beans from dry as opposed to buying canned to avoid BPA and to enjoy a better taste and texture and more nutritious and easily digestible end product. With the help of a pressure cooker, it takes no time at all. Simply soak 1 cup dry beans of choice in a bowl of filtered water overnight or for at least 6 hours. Then, drain, rinse, and add to your pressure cooker and cover completely with fresh water. Place the lid on top in the sealed position on the highest pressure for about 14 minutes, allowing for natural release. When finished, drain excess liquid and add to your favorite dish or store in an airtight container in the refrigerator for up to 5 days.

how to:
build your own
balance bowl

Choose 1-2 ingredients from each category. Bake, roast, boil, sauté, or chop and add fresh!

Greens
(1-2 cups)

Alkalizing & detoxifying
Kale, collards, spinach, chard, sprouts, herbs, romaine

Veggies
(2-3 cups)

Vitamin & mineral rich
Broccoli, tomatoes, pepper, carrots, sweet potatoes, potatoes, cabbage, cucumber, squash, beets, radish, peas, mushrooms, sauerkraut, kimchi, onion, garlic, sweet corn

Beans & Grains (& pseudo-grains)
(1 cup)

Protein & iron-rich & healthy whole food carbs
Quinoa, rice, amaranth, millet, black beans, chickpeas, lentils

Extra Protein
(½-1 cup)

Tofu, tempeh, edamame

Try it with:
Red Lentil Tofu (page 117)

Healthy Fat
(1-2 tbsp)

Rich in omega-3s for heart & brain health
Cubed avocado, hemp, chia, flax

Seasoning/Sauce
(season to taste / 1-3 tablespoons)

Added flavor and/or healthy fat
Curry powder, cumin, cinnamon, basil, oregano, nutritional yeast, coconut aminos, tamari, apple cider vinegar, balsamic, lemon, tahini, peanut butter, cilantro, lime

Try it with:
Grateful Green Guacamole (page 215), Creamy Cashew Cheeze (page 219), Perfect Pico de Gallo (page 218), Homestyle Hummus (page 213), and more from the Dips and Dressings section (page 207)

Try one of our favorite combos, the Better-for-You Burrito Bowl with Red Lentil Tofu (page 116)!

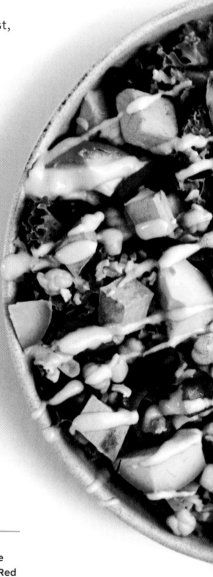

Rainbow Mango Pad Thai

This is one of my favorite raw recipes of all time, and it's so much healthier than restaurant-style pad Thai. Every color of the rainbow is present, and the sauce is to live for!

(R) | SERVES 1 TO 2 | TIME: 20 MINUTES

1 medium zucchini, unpeeled and spiralized
2 large carrots, peeled and shredded
1 red bell pepper, thinly sliced
1 cup thinly sliced red cabbage
3 green onions, thinly sliced

1 tablespoon hemp seeds
1 teaspoon sesame seeds
¾ cup shelled edamame (optional)
1 mango, diced

Sauce

1 garlic clove
¼ cup raw almond butter or peanut butter
2 tablespoons lime juice
2 tablespoons low-sodium tamari or nama shoyu

2 tablespoons filtered water
2½ teaspoons maple syrup or agave
1 teaspoon freshly grated ginger

1. In a large bowl, combine the zucchini, carrots, bell pepper, cabbage, and onions.
2. To make the sauce, place the garlic, nut butter, lime juice, tamari, water, maple syrup, and ginger in a high-speed blender and blend until smooth. Pour the mixture over the veggies and mix until well combined.
3. Sprinkle with the hemp and sesame seeds, edamame (if using), and mango and serve. Leftovers keep well in an airtight container in the refrigerator for up to 48 hours.

> **Note:** Feel free to replace the zucchini noodles with 1 (8-ounce) package of brown rice pad Thai or buckwheat soba noodles for a heartier cooked variation. You could also add our homemade Red Lentil Tofu (page 117)—cubed, marinated, and baked—to the mix.

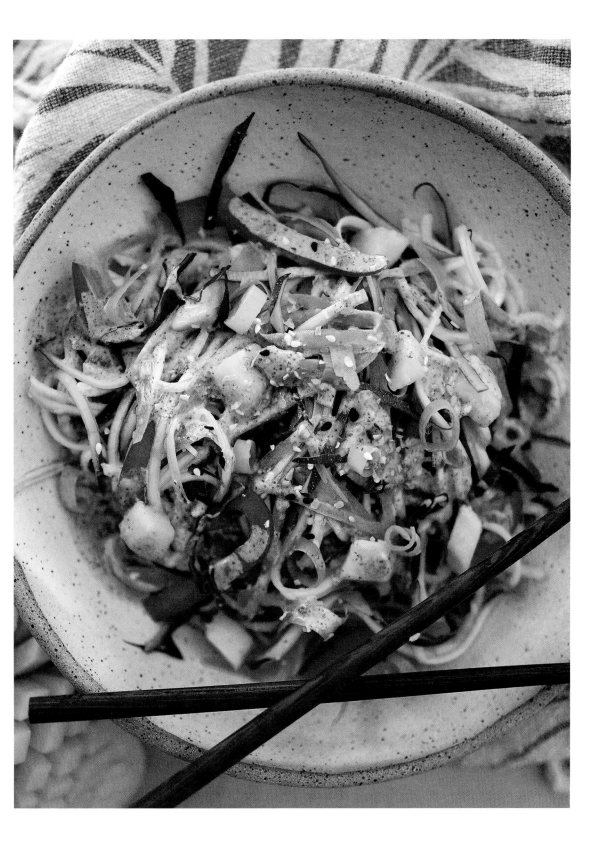

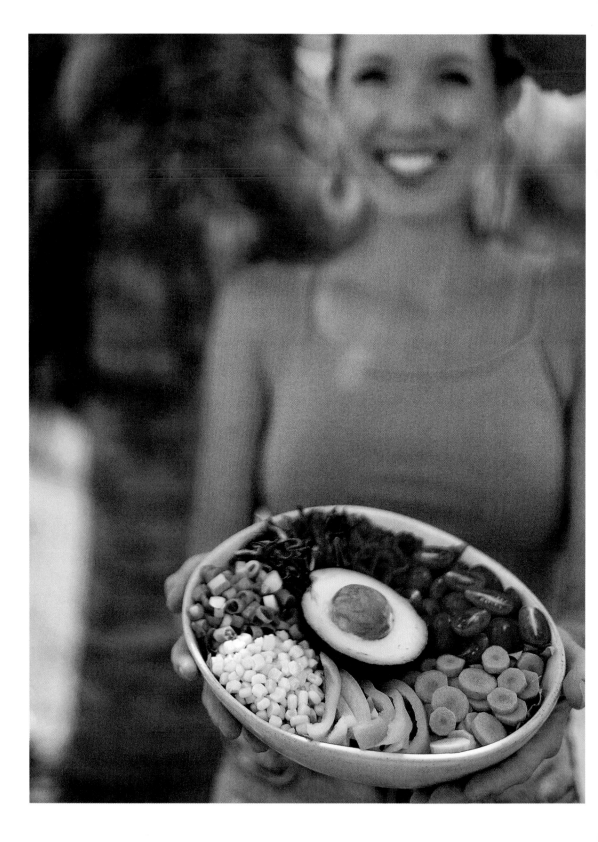

Fiesta Color Wheel Salad

This is the salad that started it all! I began making big, colorful salads when I first went plant-based, and I never looked back. My favorite part is styling this salad with every color of the rainbow and adding half an avocado for presentation. With a good mash and a twist of lime, you've got what I like to call an "un-dressing" that's easy to mix and coat your greens with, just like a dressing. You don't always need to concoct a fancy dressing to enjoy your salad, and if you're incorporating avocado, you're getting plenty of healthy fat. Make this salad your own by adding as much of your favorite veggies as you like!

(R) | SERVES 1 | TIME: 20 MINUTES

2 cups chopped leafy greens (spinach, romaine, kale, and/or arugula)

5 to 10 cherry or grape tomatoes, halved

½ cup diced orange bell pepper

1 green onion, sliced

¼ cup sweet corn kernels

Any other veggies (red cabbage, radishes, and/or carrots, etc.)

½ cup diced fresh pineapple or mango (optional)

½ avocado

2 tablespoons sauerkraut (optional)

¼ to ½ cup cooked quinoa, lentils, or beans or a handful of baked tofu (optional; for extra protein and calories)

Juice of 1 lime or lemon

Cilantro leaves, nutritional yeast, and dulse flakes, for topping (optional)

1. Place the greens in a wide and deep bowl. Top the perimeter of the bowl with the tomatoes, bell pepper, green onion, sweet corn, any other veggies, and pineapple (if using).
2. Mash or dice the avocado and mix it into the salad. Add the sauerkraut and quinoa (if using) and drizzle the lime juice on top. Mix until the greens are coated and add your choice of toppings. Best enjoyed immediately.

Superseed Everything Salad

Did you know quinoa, millet, and amaranth aren't grains? They're actually seeds, and quinoa and amaranth are complete proteins, as well. This recipe incorporates the ideal balance of raw and cooked foods as well as plenty of protein and iron, healthy fats, and carbs. It's a great recipe to make on your meal-prep day. We like to make individual portions in thirty-two-ounce mason jars, but you could also simply combine all the ingredients in one large mixing bowl, store in an airtight container in the refrigerator, and scoop out portions as needed during the week. For an added punch of flavor, top it with one of our favorite dressings, like Mason Jar Hummus Dressing.

SERVES 4 TO 6 | TIME: 20 MINUTES

½ cup quinoa

½ cup millet

½ cup amaranth

½ red onion, diced

3 garlic cloves, minced

Mason Jar Hummus Dressing (page 210)

Juice of 1 lemon

1 tablespoon nutritional yeast

1 teaspoon sea salt

Freshly ground black pepper to taste

1 cup cooked chickpeas

1 red bell pepper, diced

2 carrots, peeled and diced

½ cup frozen peas, thawed

½ cup purple cabbage, diced

1 cup fresh arugula or spinach leaves

½ avocado, diced (optional)

Sprinkle of hemp, sunflower, and/or pumpkin seeds (optional)

Handful of fresh herbs (cilantro, basil), chopped (optional)

1. Rinse the quinoa, millet, and amaranth and boil in 3 cups of filtered water for about 15 minutes or until the water is absorbed. Fluff with a fork.
2. Meanwhile, in a medium frying pan over medium heat, sauté the onion and garlic in a splash of water for 5 to 7 minutes or until the onion is translucent.
3. In a large bowl, combine the quinoa, millet, and amaranth with the onions and garlic. In four to six thirty-two-ounce mason jars, evenly distribute the Mason Jar Hummus Dressing, lemon juice, nutritional yeast, salt, and pepper and mix with a fork. Then, layer on the quinoa, millet, and amaranth mix, followed by the chickpeas, bell pepper, carrots, peas, and cabbage, and top with the arugula. Eat immediately or screw the lid on the jar and store in the refrigerator. Enjoy by pouring the salad into a large bowl and mixing well. Top it with fresh diced avocado and a sprinkle of hemp seeds and chopped herbs (if using). Leftovers can be stored in an airtight container in the refrigerator for up to 3 days.

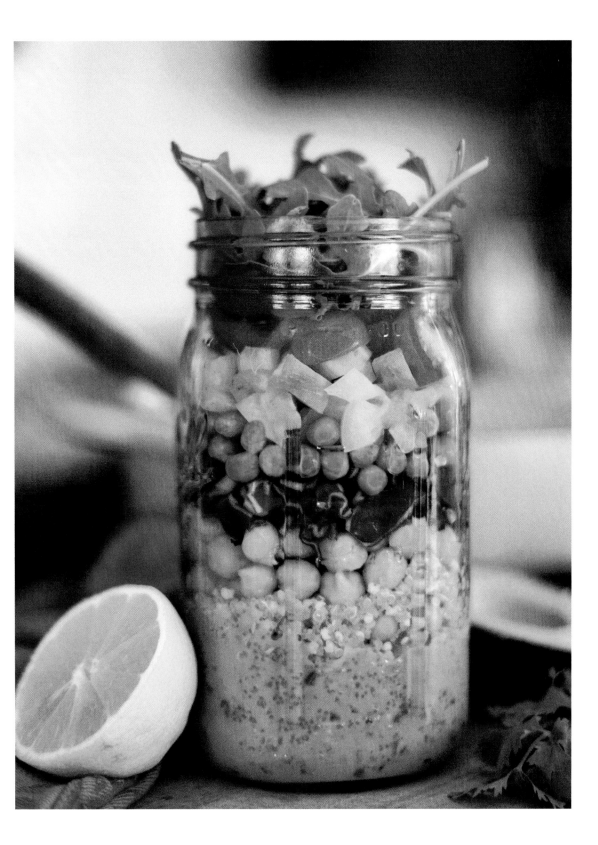

Creamy Kale & Sweet Potato Salad with Toasted Chickpeas

This salad is bursting with different colors, flavors, and textures that are sure to satisfy any craving you might have! Plus, it's easy to batch prep individual components at the beginning of the week.

SERVES 3 TO 4 | TIME: 30 MINUTES

1 (14-ounce) brick extra-firm tofu, cubed, or ½ brick of Red Lentil Tofu (page 117)
A generous drizzle of coconut aminos
2 or 3 medium sweet potatoes, cubed
1 (15.5 ounce) can chickpeas, drained and rinsed
Sea salt and freshly ground black pepper to taste

2 curly kale leaves, destemmed
¼ cup red cabbage or other raw veggies of choice, chopped
Diced avocado, sauerkraut, and nutritional yeast, for topping (optional)

Dressing Options
Creamy Cashew
½ cup raw cashews
2 tablespoons nutritional yeast

Sea salt and freshly ground black pepper to taste

Tahini Lemon
¼ cup raw tahini

Juice of 2 lemons

1. Preheat the oven to 400°F. Line three baking sheets with parchment paper.
2. In a large mixing bowl, combine the cubed tofu and coconut aminos. Toss to coat evenly and allow to marinate for at least 5 minutes (the longer the better).
3. Spread the tofu in an even layer on one of the prepared baking sheets. Bake for 15 to 20 minutes, tossing halfway through.
4. Place the sweet potatoes on a prepared baking sheet and bake for 16 to 18 minutes, tossing halfway through.
5. Pat the chickpeas dry on a kitchen towel. Spread the chickpeas in an even layer on a prepared baking sheet. Season with salt and pepper to taste. Bake for 45 minutes, mixing and tossing every 15 minutes. Watch closely to avoid burning during the final 10 minutes.
6. In a large bowl, massage the kale by tearing it into pieces and squeezing between your hands.
7. Top the kale with the tofu, sweet potato, cabbage, and your toppings of choice. (Avocado, a forkful of sauerkraut, and a dusting of nutritional yeast is the best flavor combo.)
8. Make one of the dressings: For the creamy cashew dressing, add the cashews to a mini blender with enough filtered water to cover them and allow to soak for 5 to 10 minutes. Drain and rinse. Return the cashews to the blender and cover them with filtered water. Add the nutritional yeast, salt, and pepper and blend until smooth. For the tahini lemon dressing, in a small bowl, whisk

together the tahini and lemon juice. Drizzle the dressing on top of the kale salad and dig in! Leftover sweet potatoes and chickpeas keep best in an airtight container in the refrigerator for up to 3 days.

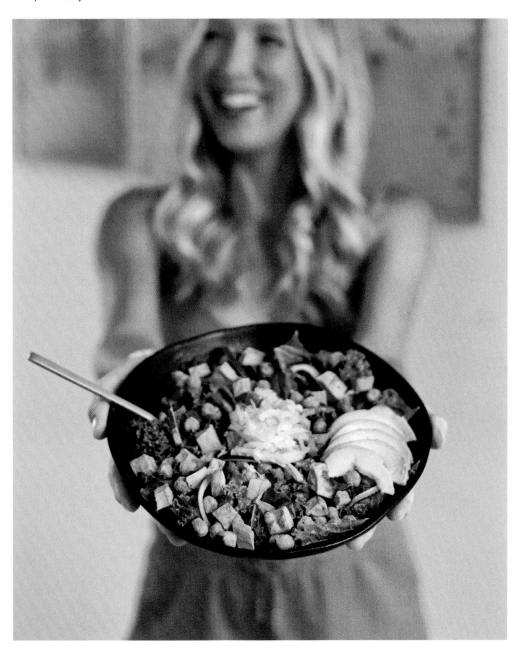

Pineapple (Un)fried Rice

This is our deliciously guilt-free take on Chinese carryout! Not only is it oil-free, it's got pineapple for extra flair! Goes great with a side of baked tofu.

(K) | SERVES 4 TO 6 | TIME: 30 MINUTES

Sea salt to taste

2 cups uncooked brown rice, rinsed, or cauliflower rice (a low-calorie option)

1 red onion, diced

3 garlic cloves, minced

1 tablespoon freshly grated ginger

Freshly ground black pepper to taste

3 carrots, peeled and diced

1 cup frozen peas, thawed

3 green onions, sliced

2 cups chopped pineapple

Coconut aminos, tamari, or soy sauce to taste

1. Bring 4½ cups filtered water to a boil with a pinch of salt. Add the brown rice, reduce the heat to medium-low, and cook until tender and the water is absorbed, about 20 minutes.
2. Add a splash of water to a medium sauté pan over medium-high heat and sauté the onion, garlic, and ginger with salt and pepper for 5 minutes. Add the carrots and sauté until they are fork-tender.
3. In a large bowl, combine the rice, carrot mixture, peas, green onions, and pineapple.
4. Dish up and drizzle with coconut aminos. Leftovers keep well in an airtight container in the refrigerator for up to 3 days.

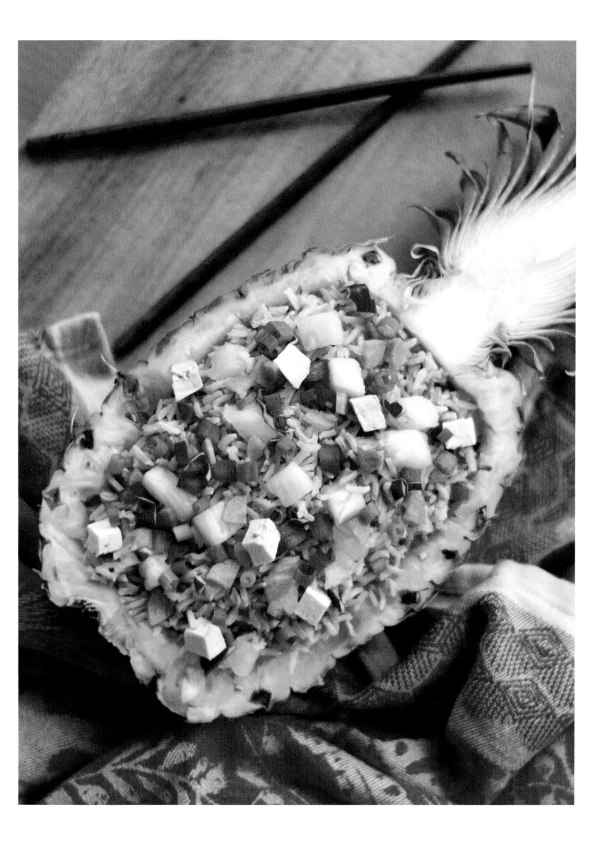

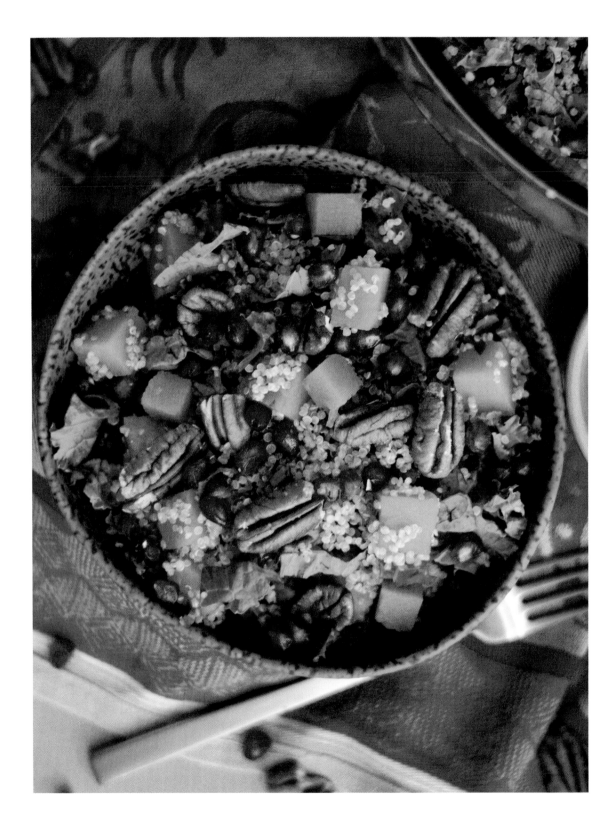

Butternut Squash Pomegranate Quinoa Salad

This recipe is bursting with color and flavor and boasts a wide range of nutrients, including complete protein in the quinoa, vitamin A in the squash, and loads of antioxidants thanks to the pomegranate. It's something fresh that you can enjoy even in the dead of winter and it's great for bringing to holiday gatherings, as well!

SERVES 4 | TIME: 30 MINUTES

2 to 3 cups cubed butternut squash
1 cup quinoa, rinsed
3 cups shredded lacinato (dinosaur) or curly kale leaves, destemmed, plus more to taste
½ cup pomegranate arils
½ cup raw pecans

1 teaspoon apple cider vinegar
¼ cup raw tahini
1½ tablespoons maple syrup
Sea salt and freshly ground black pepper to taste
Nutritional yeast to taste (optional)

1. Preheat the oven to 400°F. Line a baking sheet with parchment paper.
2. Spread the squash in an even layer on the prepared baking sheet and sprinkle with water. Roast for 30 minutes, stirring after 15 minutes.
3. While the squash is roasting, add the quinoa to a medium pot with 2 cups filtered water. Bring to a boil, reduce the heat to medium-low, and simmer for 15 minutes or until the water is absorbed. Remove from the heat and fluff with a fork.
4. In a large mixing bowl, combine the cooled quinoa and squash, kale, pomegranates, and pecans.
5. To make the dressing, in a small bowl whisk together the apple cider vinegar, tahini, and maple syrup until smooth and creamy. If it's too thick, add a splash of water to thin it out a bit.
6. Drizzle the dressing on top of the salad or serve it on the side. Add salt, pepper, and nutritional yeast (if using) on top for added flavor. Leftovers keep best in an airtight container in the refrigerator for up to 3 days. Consider adding additional fresh kale to each dish when plating to eat.

Sushi Bowls with Baked Tofu

These bowls will fill you up and nourish your body more than your run-of-the-mill sushi roll will!

SERVES 2 | TIME: 30 MINUTES

1 (14-ounce) block extra-firm tofu, cubed, or ½ block of Red Lentil Tofu (page 117)

¼ cup coconut aminos

Sea salt to taste

1 cup uncooked short grain brown rice or ½ head cauliflower, riced

1 carrot, shredded

1 red bell pepper, thinly sliced

1 cucumber, thinly sliced

1 cup frozen shelled edamame or peas, thawed

2 green onions, chopped

½ cup sliced purple cabbage

1 avocado, diced

Handful of microgreens or sprouts (optional)

Sauce

1 to 2 tablespoons coconut aminos

¼ cup peanut or almond butter

Juice of ½ lime (optional)

1. Preheat the oven to 400°F. Line a baking sheet with parchment paper.
2. To a large mixing bowl, add the tofu and coconut aminos. Toss to coat evenly and allow to marinate for at least 5 minutes (the longer the better).
3. Spread the tofu in an even layer on the prepared baking sheet. Bake for 15 to 20 minutes, tossing halfway through.
4. In a large pot, bring 2 cups filtered water to a boil with a pinch of salt. Add the brown rice, reduce the heat to medium-low, and cook until fluffy and the water is absorbed, about 20 minutes.
5. In a large bowl, arrange the rice, tofu, carrot, bell pepper, cucumber, edamame, green onions, cabbage, avocado, and microgreens (if using).
6. To make the sauce, mix the coconut aminos with the nut butter and lime juice (if using). Add 1 tablespoon filtered water to achieve a thinner consistency.
7. To serve, drizzle the sauce on top and enjoy with chopsticks . . . if you're up for the challenge! Leftovers keep best in an airtight container in the refrigerator for up to 3 days.

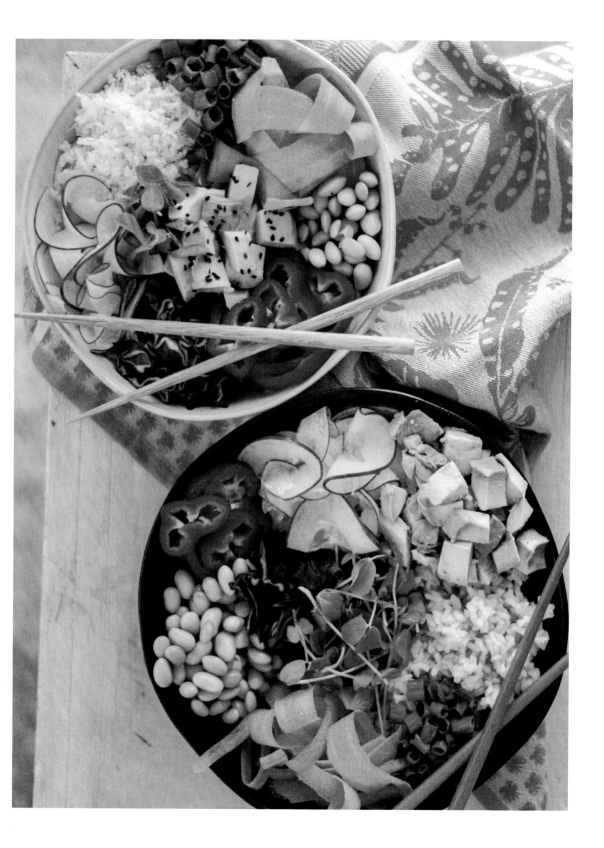

Sandwiches & Wraps

No utensils required in this section! We've taken all our favorite colorful raw and cooked combos and sandwiched them into some epic meals. This section is where you can get creative, sneaking in some extra nutritious ingredients that you or your little ones might otherwise shy away from. The Bountiful Black Bean Veggie Burgers (page 141) are a perfect example of how you can pack a powerful punch while still feeling like you're enjoying your favorite classic burger.

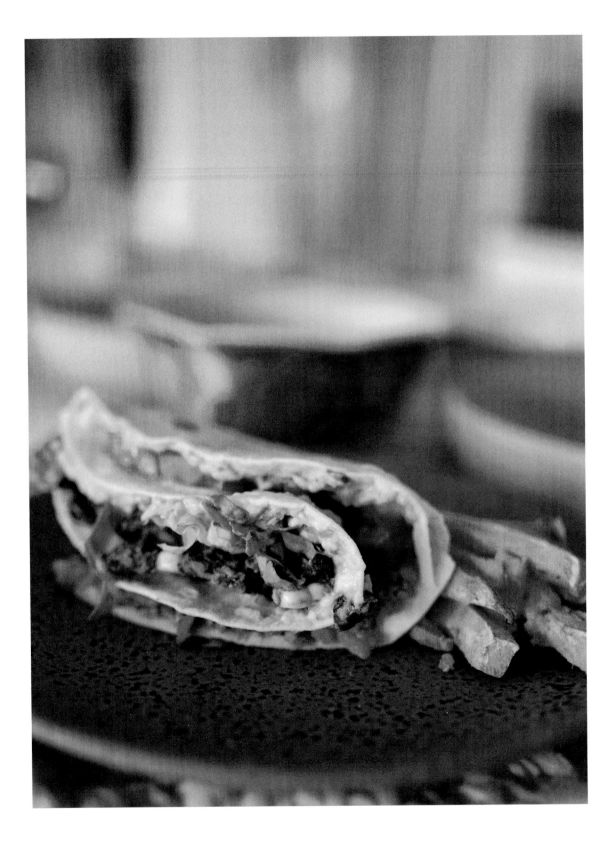

Taco-Bout Tasty Fold-Up

It tastes like a taco from your favorite drive-through, but this little handheld triangle of deliciousness is way more nutritious! Feel free to get creative and pile in other ingredients to make a combo all your own. Round it out with a side of sweet potato fries.

(DIY) (K) | SERVES 1 | TIME: 10 MINUTES

1 whole wheat tortilla

1 tablespoon Homestyle Hummus (page 213) or Creamy Cashew Cheeze (page 219)

¼ cup cooked quinoa, brown rice, or green lentils

1 tablespoon mashed avocado or Grateful Green Guacamole (page 215), plus more for serving

Handful of shredded romaine lettuce or spinach leaves

¼ cup lack beans or chickpeas, smashed

Nutritional yeast to taste

Sea salt and freshly ground black pepper to taste

Taco sauce, sriracha sauce, or salsa, for dipping (optional)

1. Lay the tortilla flat and make a cut from the center, outward to the bottom edge.
2. Envision four quadrants on your tortilla. Spread hummus on the bottom left quadrant. Sprinkle quinoa on the top left quadrant. Spread avocado topped with lettuce on the top right quadrant. Spread the beans on the bottom right quadrant.
3. Sprinkle the nutritional yeast, salt, and pepper on top and begin folding over. Start with the bottom left hummus quadrant and fold up and around.
4. In a small frying pan over medium-low heat, cook the fold-up for 2 to 3 minutes on each side, or until crisp and golden brown. Try dipped in taco sauce (if desired) or additional guacamole. Best enjoyed immediately or wrapped in tinfoil for on-the-go.

Colorful Collard Wraps

These wraps are bursting with flavor and color from a handful of juicy and crisp raw foods, such as carrot, cucumber, bell pepper, cabbage, and mango. It's also a fun and effortless way to go fork-free with your salads!

(R) | SERVES 1 | TIME: 15 MINUTES

1 or 2 large collard leaves

1 tablespoon Homestyle Hummus (page 213) or Grateful Green Guacamole (page 215)

1 carrot, thinly sliced

1 cucumber, thinly sliced

1 red bell pepper, thinly sliced

½ cup purple cabbage, thinly sliced

¼ mango, thinly sliced

¼ avocado, thinly sliced

Handful of sprouts

Tropical Mango Salad Dressing (page 221) or Rainbow Mango Pad Thai sauce (page 120), for dipping (optional)

1. Flip each collard leaf onto its back side and shave off the top "ridge" of the stem to make the leaf easier to roll without breaking.
2. Spread the hummus on a collard leaf and place in the middle of the leaf a thin layer of carrot, cucumber, bell pepper, cabbage, mango, avocado, and sprouts on top. Begin to wrap at one end, folding the edges in, and continue to roll up all the way.
3. Slice the wrap in half and enjoy as is, or try dipping it in Tropical Mango Salad Dressing or the Rainbow Mango Pad Thai sauce. Best enjoyed immediately or wrapped in tinfoil for on-the-go.

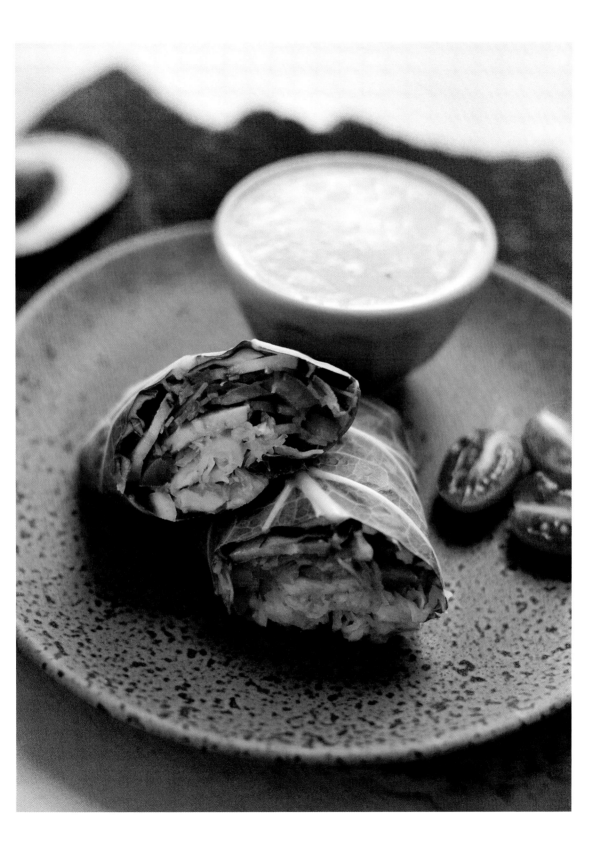

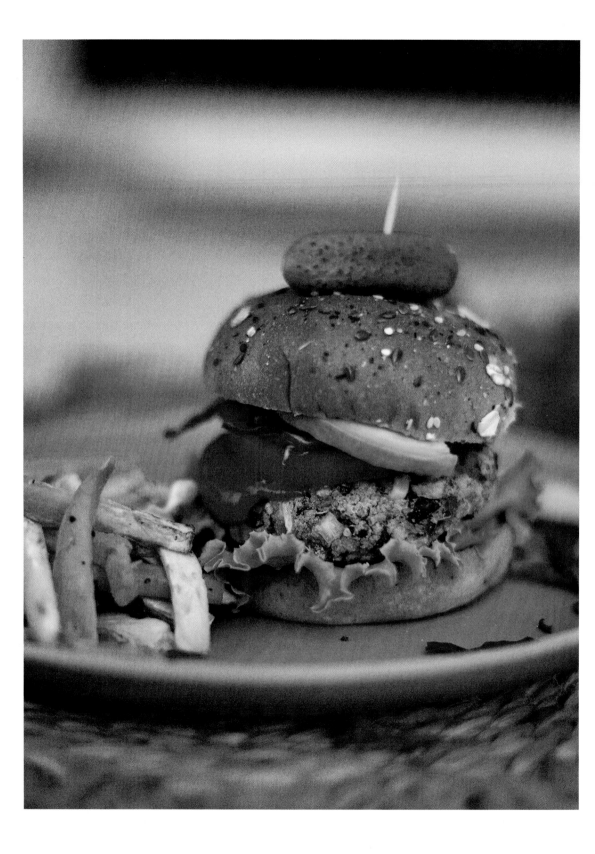

Bountiful Black Bean Veggie Burgers

These burgers are loaded with plant protein and plenty of flavor! We love making veggie burgers with family and friends when we can be outside using the grill, and they're a fun finger food for kiddos. Pair them with a side of baked potato wedges or sweet potato fries.

MAKES 12 TO 14 BURGERS | TIME: 45 MINUTES

2 (15.5 ounce) cans black beans, drained and rinsed

2 cups cooked quinoa

2 medium tomatoes, diced

1 cup diced red onion

½ cup sweet corn kernels (optional)

1 medium carrot, shredded

2 garlic cloves, minced

1 cup brown rice or oat flour

1 tablespoon hot sauce (we like sriracha)

1 teaspoon ground cumin

Sea salt and freshly ground black pepper to taste

12 to 14 hamburger buns (Ezekiel, whole wheat, or gluten-free)

Avocado, green-leaf lettuce, red onion, tomato, pickles, and ketchup, for topping (optional)

1. Preheat the oven to 350°F. Line a baking sheet with parchment paper.
2. Place the beans in a large mixing bowl and smash with a fork. Add the quinoa, tomatoes, onion, corn (if using), carrot, garlic, flour, hot sauce, cumin, salt, and pepper and mix with your hands until well combined.
3. Use your hands to scoop ½ cup of the bean mixture, form into a ball, and flatten onto the prepared baking sheet, creating patties about ½-inch thick. Repeat until you've used all the mixture.
4. Bake the patties for 15 minutes on each side. (Or on a grill, cook on the baking sheet for 5 to 7 minutes on each side, or until cooked to your liking.)
5. Serve the burgers on the buns with your choice of toppings! Patties can be stored in an airtight container in the refrigerator for up to 3 days or in the freezer for up to a month.

Chickpea Falafel Patties

These patties are the perfect punch of plant protein! They're super flavorful thanks to a few key spices, and they can be made into large patties for sandwiches or bite-size for dipping.

MAKES 9 OR 10 PATTIES | TIME: 35 MINUTES

1 (15.5-ounce) can chickpeas, drained and rinsed
½ cup rolled oats
1 medium sweet potato, cooked
2 cups fresh spinach leaves
¼ cup fresh parsley
2 tablespoons nutritional yeast
1 tablespoon raw tahini
1 tablespoon ground flaxseeds

1 teaspoon ground cumin
1 teaspoon garlic powder
½ teaspoon onion powder
Sea salt and freshly ground black pepper to taste
9 or 10 buns (Ezekiel, whole wheat, or gluten-free)
Avocado or guacamole, leafy greens (arugula, spinach), and red cabbage, for topping (optional)

1. Preheat the oven to 350°F. Line a baking sheet with parchment paper.
2. To a food processor, add the chickpeas, oats, sweet potato, spinach, parsley, nutritional yeast, tahini, flaxseeds, cumin, garlic powder, onion powder, salt, and pepper. Process until all the ingredients are well combined.
3. Use your hands to scoop ½ cup of the chickpea mixture, form into a ball, and flatten onto the baking sheet, creating patties about ½-inch thick. Repeat until you've used all the mixture. Bake in the oven for 20 minutes, flipping halfway through.
4. Allow the patties to cool for about 10 minutes before serving on the buns with the toppings of your choice. Patties can be stored in an airtight container in the refrigerator for up to 3 days or in the freezer for up to a month.

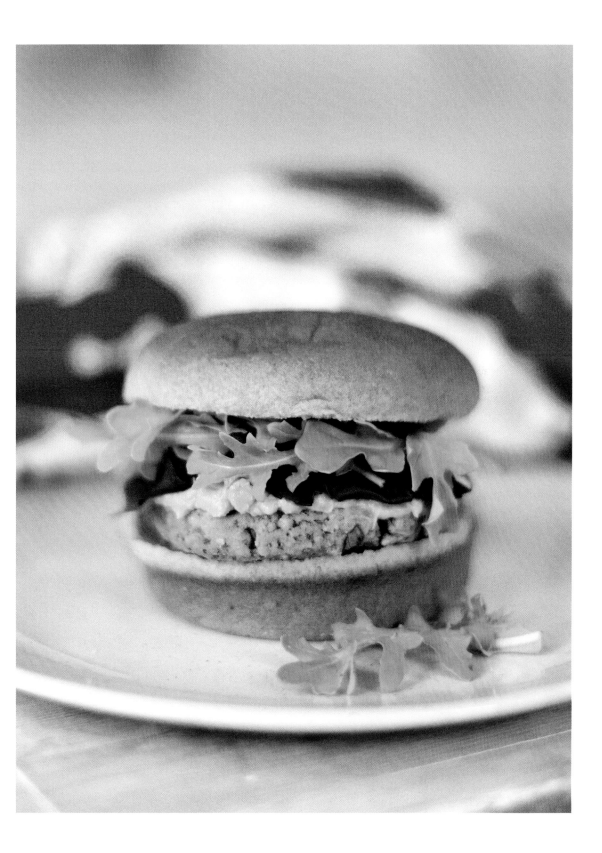

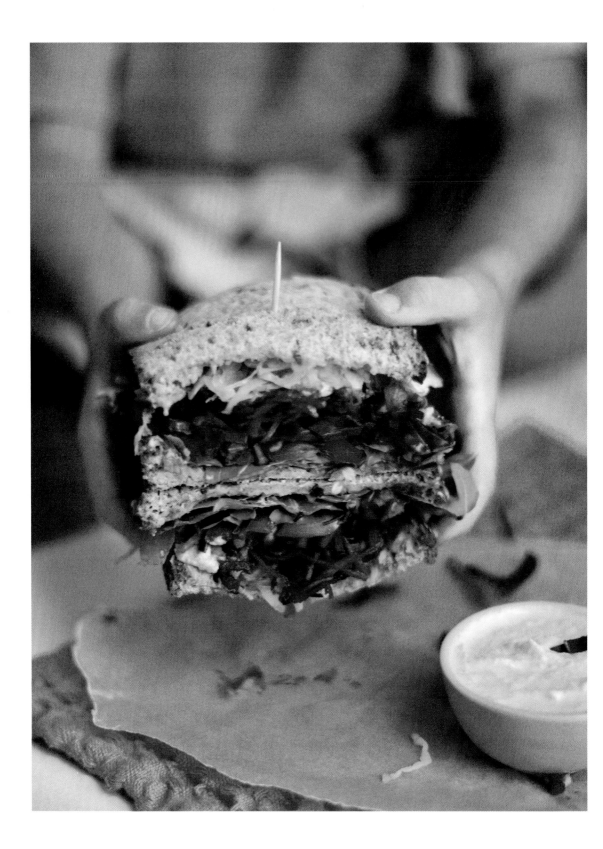

Stacked Veggie Sandwich

Whatever happened to the lost art of creating a tasty homemade sandwich?! No need to reinvent the wheel, just add only plants and leave out the mayo and lunch meat! We love bringing these to the beach or the park for a picnic!

SERVES 1 | TIME: 10 MINUTES

2 slices sprouted whole wheat or gluten-free bread (see Note below)
1 tablespoon Homestyle Hummus (page 213)
¼ avocado, mashed
2 leaves green-leaf lettuce
3 slices tomato

5 thin slices yellow bell pepper
2 tablespoons shredded beet
2 tablespoons shredded carrot
1 tablespoon sauerkraut
Sprinkle of nutritional yeast
Sea salt and freshly ground black pepper to taste

1. Toast the bread and start building your sandwich.
2. Spread the hummus on one slice of the bread and the avocado on the other. Add the lettuce, tomato, bell pepper, beet, carrot, sauerkraut, nutritional yeast, salt, and pepper and close up. Slice in half and open wide! Best enjoyed immediately or wrapped in tinfoil to take on-the-go.

Note: We love Ezekiel bread because it contains all essential amino acids from six organically grown, sprouted whole grains and legumes. If you can't find that option, look for bread that contains organic whole wheat as the first ingredient and does not contain added sugar or oil.

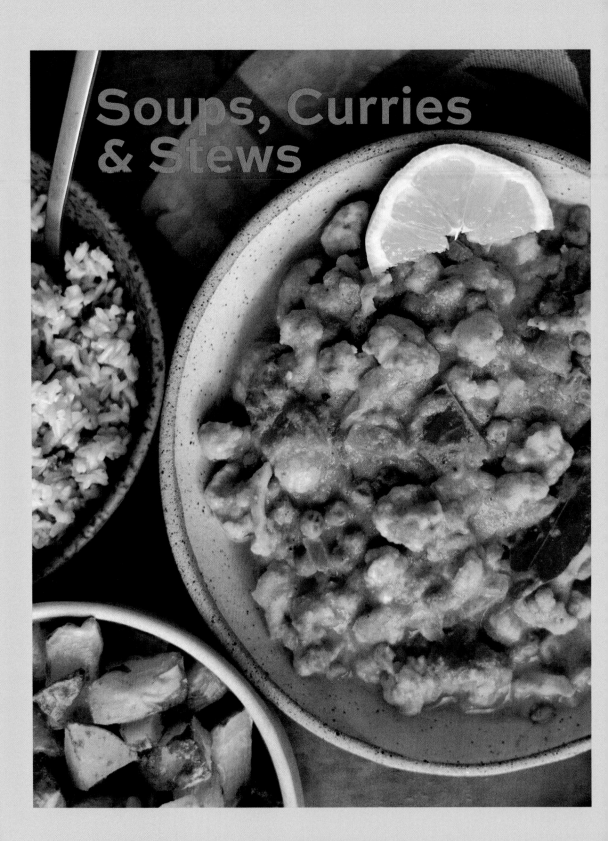

Soups, Curries
& Stews

Our giant, bright blue Dutch oven is a staple we couldn't live without. We like to cook up a massive soup, curry, or stew that will get us through two dinners so we don't have to cook every single night. With the right herbs and spices, many versatile and otherwise bland plant foods come to life in so many different, delicious variations. Get ready for loads of lentils, a bounty of beans, the right amount of rice, and a variety of veggies!

Coconut Quinoa Yellow Curry

This dish tastes just like one we loved to order at Thai restaurants, and the quinoa adds a complete protein.

(K) | SERVES 4 TO 6 | TIME: 45 MINUTES

1 yellow onion, diced

3 or 4 garlic cloves, minced

3 to 4 cups vegetable broth (depending on how thick you'd like your curry to be), plus more for the pan

1 teaspoon ground coriander

1 teaspoon ground turmeric

1 teaspoon curry powder

1 teaspoon chopped fresh cilantro leaves

2 tablespoons yellow curry paste

Sea salt and freshly ground black pepper to taste

1½ cups quinoa, rinsed

4 to 5 unpeeled carrots, chopped

½ to 1 whole cauliflower, depending on size

3 medium sweet potatoes, peeled and chopped

1½ cups frozen peas

2 medium tomatoes, chopped

¼ cup unsweetened coconut milk or cream

Dash of red pepper flakes (optional)

Jasmine or brown basmati rice, for serving

1. In a large pot over medium heat, sauté the onion and garlic in a splash of vegetable broth and cook until the onion is translucent. Add the coriander, turmeric, curry powder, cilantro, curry paste, salt, and pepper and continue to sauté for 2 to 3 minutes, until fragrant.

2. Add the vegetable broth, quinoa, carrots, cauliflower, and sweet potatoes, bring to a boil over medium-high heat, reduce back to medium heat, and cook for 15 to 20 minutes, or until the root veggies are soft.

3. Add the frozen peas, tomatoes, and coconut milk and continue to cook for 2 to 3 more minutes.

4. Divide the curry among individual bowls and season to your liking with salt, pepper, and red pepper flakes (if using). Serve with a side of rice. Leftovers keep best in an airtight container in the refrigerator for up to 3 days.

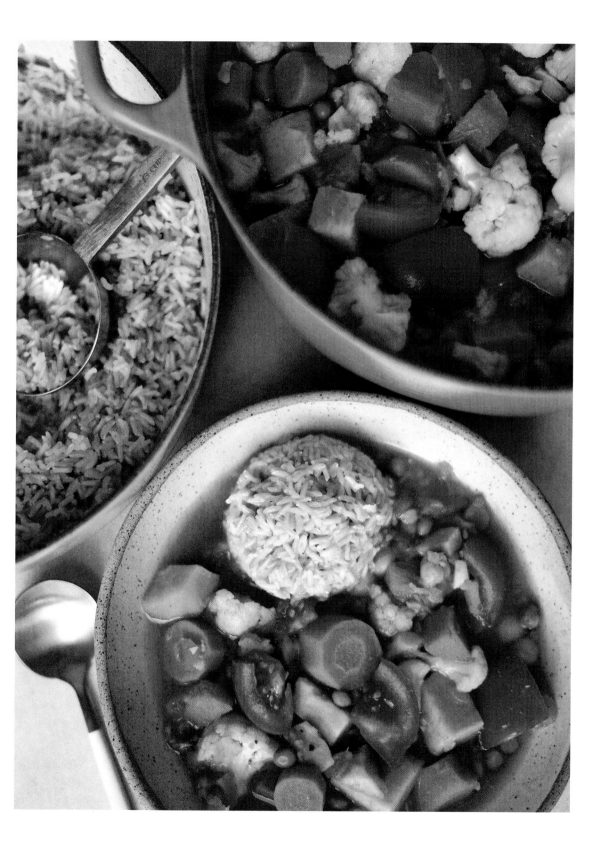

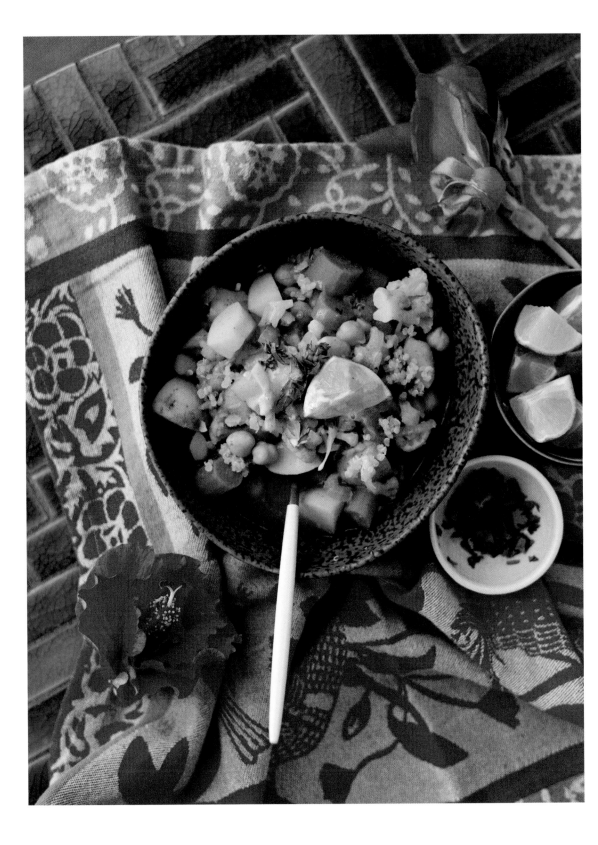

Quinoa Veggie Immunity Soup

This is a total "mom" recipe. I grew up enjoying some variation of this soup whenever I was feeling under the weather. The natural flavor combination of the veggies truly shines through in this effortless, cozy soup.

SERVES 4 TO 6 | TIME: 45 MINUTES

1 sweet yellow onion, diced

3 or 4 garlic cloves, minced

½-inch piece fresh ginger, unpeeled and grated

3 medium unpeeled carrots, sliced

3 celery stalks, sliced

2 bay leaves

Sea salt and freshly ground black pepper to taste

1 cup quinoa, rinsed

4 cups vegetable broth

2 large sweet potatoes or russet potatoes, chopped (or one of each)

1 red bell pepper, diced

½ cup diced mushrooms

½ teaspoon ground turmeric

1 teaspoon curry powder

1 (15.5-ounce) can chickpeas, drained and rinsed (optional)

1 cup shredded kale

Nutritional yeast to taste

1. In a large pot with a splash of water, sauté the onion, garlic, ginger, carrots, and celery over medium heat until the onion is translucent and carrots are fork-tender. Add the bay leaves and season with salt and pepper.
2. Add the quinoa, vegetable broth, sweet potatoes, bell pepper, mushrooms, turmeric, and curry powder and bring to a boil. Cover, reduce to medium-low heat, and simmer until the veggies are fork-tender.
3. Add the chickpeas (if using) and cook for an additional 5 minutes.
4. Remove from the heat and stir in the kale.
5. Serve with a dusting of nutritional yeast for an added boost of flavor and nutrition. Leftovers keep best in an airtight container in the refrigerator for up to 3 days.

Creamy Cashew Cauliflower Curry & Air-Fried Spiced Potatoes

We were sparked to create this dish by one of our favorite chefs, Richa Hingle (Vegan Richa), who creates flavorful recipes inspired by her Indian roots. Savory, rich, creamy, slightly sweet, not too spicy, and seasoned to perfection, this curry is the one we make when there is something to celebrate in our household. The sauce is out of this world!

SERVES 4 | TIME: 40 MINUTES

1 cup uncooked brown basmati rice, rinsed

5 or 6 medium Yukon Gold potatoes, cubed

2 teaspoons sea salt or to taste

Freshly ground black pepper to taste

1 teaspoon curry powder

1 teaspoon cumin seeds or ½ teaspoon ground cumin

1 bay leaf

½ red onion, diced

2 medium tomatoes, chopped

¼ cup raw cashews, soaked 3 hours, drained, and rinsed

3 garlic cloves, minced

1-inch piece fresh ginger, unpeeled and grated

1 teaspoon garam masala

½ teaspoon ground coriander

½ teaspoon ground mustard

½ teaspoon cayenne pepper (optional)

½ teaspoon ground turmeric

¼ teaspoon ground cinnamon

1 head cauliflower, cut into small florets

¾ cup frozen peas

Fresh cilantro leaves and lemon wedges, for garnish

1. In a large pot, place the rice with 2 cups filtered water. Bring to a boil and reduce the heat to low. Cover, with the lid slightly cracked, and allow to simmer. Cook about 25 minutes, stirring occasionally, until the liquid is almost completely absorbed. Fluff the rice with a fork, scoop into a serving dish, and cover.

2. Preheat the air fryer to 400°F. Add the potatoes to the air fryer. Dust with salt, pepper, and curry powder and toss to coat evenly. Cook for 15 to 20 minutes, tossing halfway through, until desired crispiness. Set aside.

3. In a large sauté pan over medium heat, sauté the cumin and bay leaf in a splash of water until fragrant, about 2 minutes. Add the onion and continue to sauté until cooked through.

4. To make the sauce, place the tomatoes, cashews, garlic, ginger, garam masala, coriander, mustard, cayenne (if using), turmeric, and cinnamon in a high-speed blender and blend until smooth.

5. Add the sauce to the pan, mix well, and cook for 10 minutes.

6. Add salt, ½ cup filtered water, and cauliflower, stir, cover, and simmer on medium-low for about 15 minutes or until the cauliflower is fork-tender.

7. Add the peas and season with salt, pepper, and other spices as desired. Stir to combine and then cover and cook until the peas are tender. Garnish with the cilantro and lemon and serve over basmati rice, alongside the spiced, air-fried potatoes. Leftovers keep best in an airtight container in the refrigerator for up to 3 days.

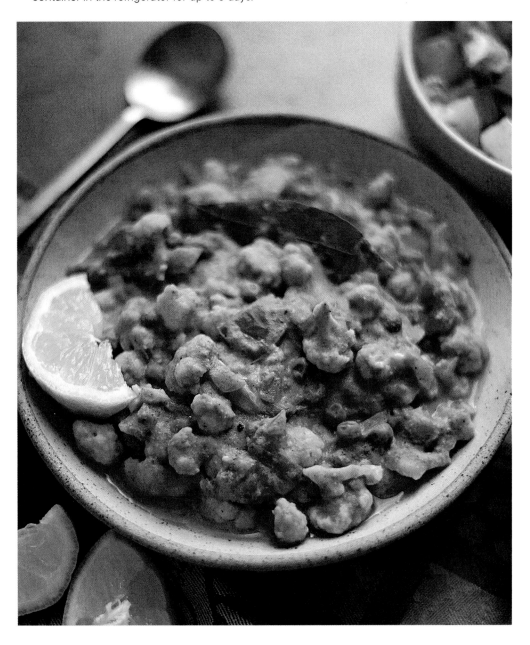

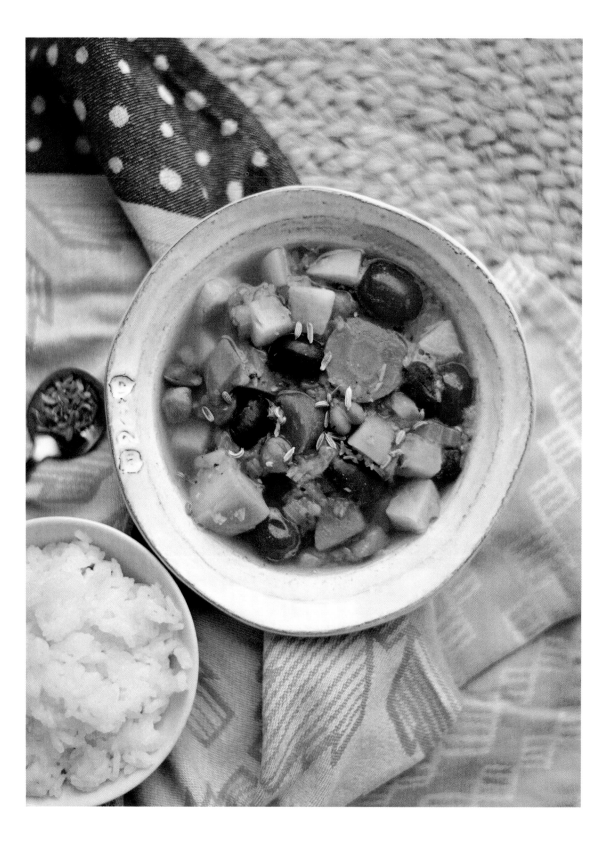

Moroccan Spice Veggie Soup

This soup is all about the spices! It has such a unique flavor profile, and it's also loaded with protein and iron thanks to the lentils and beans. The fennel and ginger are also amazing for gut health and digestion.

SERVES 6 | TIME: 1 HOUR

1 yellow onion, diced

3 or 4 garlic cloves, minced

Splash of vegetable broth

1 teaspoon cumin seeds

½ teaspoon fennel seeds

1 teaspoon ground turmeric

1 teaspoon ground coriander

¾ teaspoon ground ginger

1 teaspoon dried basil

Dash of ground cinnamon

Dash of cayenne pepper

Sea salt and freshly ground black pepper to taste

1 cup dried red lentils

2 to 3 cups peeled and cubed garnet and/or Japanese (white flesh) sweet potato

2 medium carrots, unpeeled and sliced

1 (15.5-ounce) can chickpeas, drained and rinsed

1 (15.5-ounce) can kidney beans, drained and rinsed

Handful of cherry or grape tomatoes

Jasmine or basmati rice (white or brown), for serving

Sprinkle of fennel seeds, for garnish

½ cup chopped raw peanuts, for garnish (optional)

1. In a large pot over medium heat, sauté the onion and garlic in a splash of veggie broth until the onion is translucent.
2. Add the cumin, fennel, turmeric, coriander, ginger, basil, cinnamon, cayenne, salt, and pepper and continue sautéing until fragrant, about 2 minutes.
3. Add the lentils, sweet potatoes, carrots, chickpeas, and kidney beans and cover with filtered water. Cook over medium heat until the potatoes and carrots are fork-tender.
4. Add the cherry tomatoes and cook for 5 minutes, or until they are softened.
5. Serve with a side of rice and garnish with a sprinkle of fennel seeds and optional peanuts. Leftovers keep best in an airtight container in the refrigerator for up to 3 days.

Sweet Potato & Kale Chili

This cold-weather favorite is loaded with plant protein and will make your whole house smell cozy and comforting. Leftovers go great over baked sweet potatoes for a quick and satisfying weeknight meal!

SERVES 4 TO 6 | TIME: 50 MINUTES

1 small red onion, diced
3 garlic cloves, minced
3 celery stalks, sliced
1 red, orange, or yellow bell pepper, diced
3 medium tomatoes, diced
1 (15-ounce) can diced tomatoes
2 teaspoons ground cumin
4 teaspoons dried oregano
1 cup dried green lentils
1¾ cups cooked (or 1 [15.5-ounce] can) kidney beans

1¾ cups cooked (or 1 [15.5-ounce] can) navy beans
3 medium sweet potatoes, garnet and/or Japanese (white flesh) varieties, cubed
1 teaspoon paprika
1 teaspoon chili powder
Sea salt and freshly ground black pepper to taste
1 cup sweet corn kernels
2 cups shredded kale or collards
1 avocado, cubed or sliced (optional)

1. In a medium to large pot over medium heat, simmer the onion, garlic, celery, bell pepper, fresh tomatoes, canned tomatoes, cumin, and oregano for 10 minutes. Add half of the mixture to a high-speed blender, blend until smooth, and return to the pot.
2. Add the lentils, kidney beans, navy beans, sweet potatoes, paprika, chili powder, salt, pepper, and 2 cups filtered water. Bring to a boil, reduce to medium-low heat, and cook covered for about 20 minutes, or until lentils and sweet potatoes are fork-tender.
3. Add the sweet corn and kale and cook for another 2 to 3 minutes, or until the kale turns dark green.
4. Serve with sliced avocado on top! Leftovers keep best in an airtight container in the refrigerator for up to 3 days.

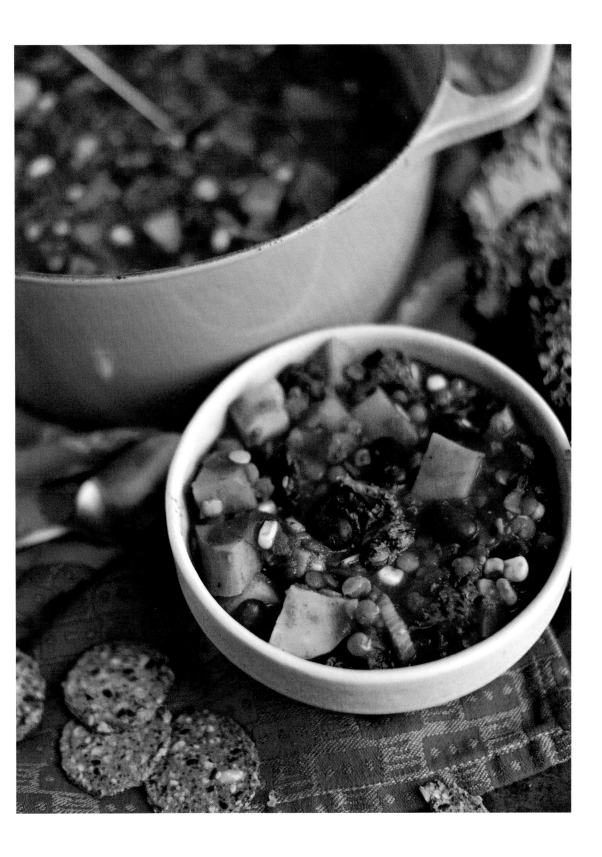

Root Veggie Stew

This is the first plant-based dinner that we fell in love with, and we still make it routinely! The beets give this dish a deep red color and a slightly sweet taste. A fall favorite that pairs well with this meal is roasted Brussels sprouts. Be sure to include your favorite sourdough or gluten-free bread for dipping, as well!

SERVES 4 TO 6 | TIME: 50 MINUTES

1 large sweet onion, diced

2 garlic cloves, minced

½-inch piece fresh ginger, unpeeled and minced (optional)

4 cups liquid (filtered water, vegetable broth, and/or unsweetened coconut milk)

1 cup dried red lentils, rinsed

3 or 4 sweet potatoes, cubed (about 6 cups)

3 medium beets, cubed

4 carrots, unpeeled and thinly sliced

4 celery stalks, thinly sliced

3 curly kale leaves, destemmed

Sea salt and freshly ground black pepper to taste

1. In a large pot over medium heat, add a splash of water and sauté the onion, garlic, and ginger (if using) until translucent.
2. Add the liquid and red lentils. Bring to a boil, reduce the heat to medium-low, and add the sweet potatoes, beets, carrots, celery, and kale. Stir well, cover, and simmer until the root veggies are soft.
3. Season with salt and pepper to taste and serve. Leftovers keep best in an airtight container in the refrigerator for up to 3 days.

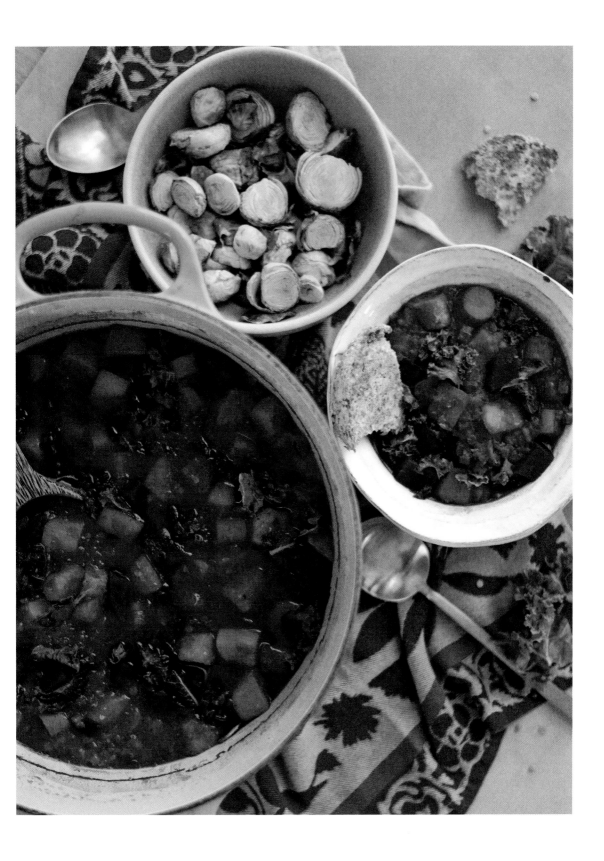

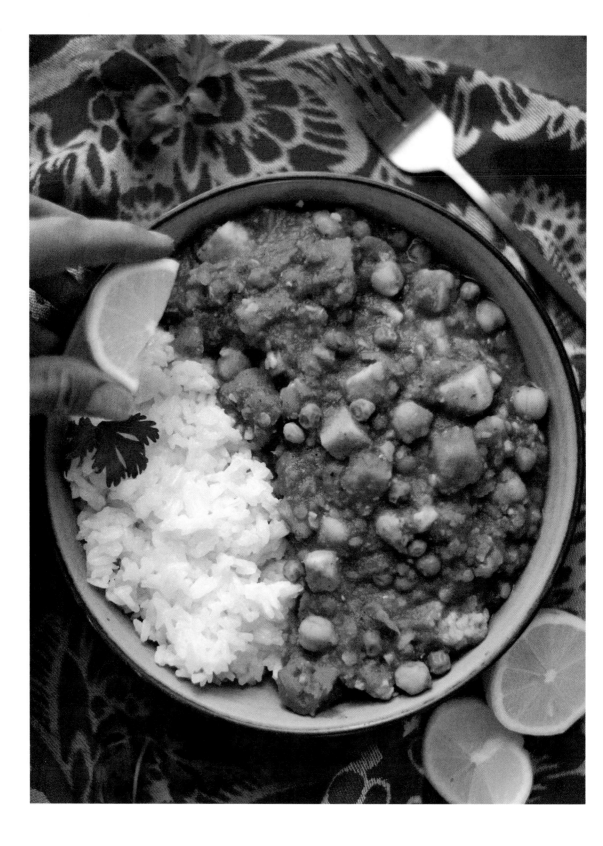

Curry Spiced Red Lentil Stew

This stew is perfectly spiced! We typically start it in the morning and let it cook low and slow in a slow cooker all day, to bring out the most flavor, but you can also cook it on the stovetop in about forty-five minutes. This is a recipe we especially like to make when we are feeling super busy and need something hearty and filling to come home to that keeps us full and extra nourished.

SERVES 4 TO 6 | TIME: 4 TO 8 HOURS

2 cups dried red lentils

2 sweet potatoes, cubed

1 large sweet onion, diced

2 garlic cloves, minced

1 large head cauliflower, cut into small florets

1 (15.5-ounce) can chickpeas, drained and rinsed

1 cup frozen peas, thawed

2 tablespoons red curry paste

1 tablespoon minced fresh ginger

1 (28-ounce) can tomato puree

1 teaspoon ground turmeric

½ teaspoon ground coriander

½ teaspoon ground cumin

½ teaspoon cayenne pepper

¼ teaspoon ground cardamom

Sea salt and freshly ground black pepper to taste

1½ cups filtered water

Fresh cilantro leaves and lemon wedges, for garnish

1. Add the lentils to the bottom of a slow cooker. Top with the sweet potatoes and then the onion, garlic, cauliflower, chickpeas, peas, curry paste, ginger, tomato puree, turmeric, coriander, cumin, cayenne pepper, cardamom, salt, pepper, and filtered water.
2. Cover and cook on high for 4 to 5 hours or low for 7 to 8 hours.
3. Enjoy garnished with cilantro and a lemon wedge. Leftovers keep best in an airtight container in the refrigerator for up to 3 days.

Ramen & Veggies

This is one of our go-to, quick-and-easy lunch recipes that the kids love. Noodles will always win over even the most selective eaters, and the colorful veggies add so much nutrition and flavor. Feel free to get creative and add in your favorite veggies and seasonings!

SERVES 2 | TIME: 15 MINUTES

2 packs rice or buckwheat ramen

2 tablespoons miso paste

1 tablespoon tamari or liquid aminos

½ teaspoon garlic powder

½ teaspoon onion powder

1 (14-ounce) block firm tofu, cubed, or Red Lentil Tofu (page 117)

1 medium carrot, shredded

1 cup broccoli florets

½ cup sliced mushrooms

½ cup frozen shelled edamame or lima beans (optional)

Sea salt and freshly ground black pepper to taste

Thinly sliced red cabbage, thinly sliced bok choi, chopped green onion, dulse flakes, and/or red pepper flakes, for topping

1. In a medium to large pot, bring 4 cups filtered water to a boil, add the ramen, and reduce the heat to medium. Add the miso paste, tamari, garlic powder, onion powder, tofu, carrot, broccoli, mushrooms, and edamame (if using). Season with salt and pepper to taste.

2. When the noodles are tender, serve in bowls with your choice of toppings. Leftovers keep best in an airtight container in the refrigerator for up to 3 days.

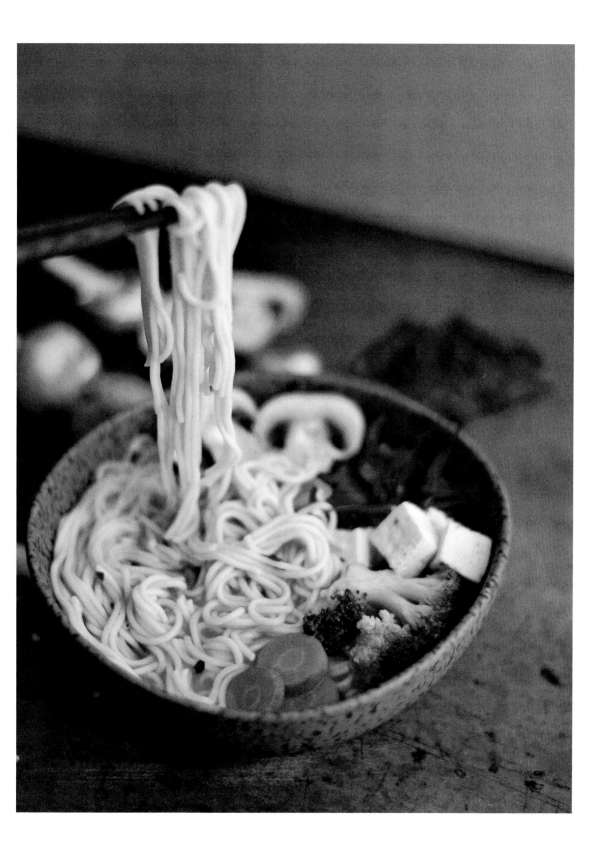

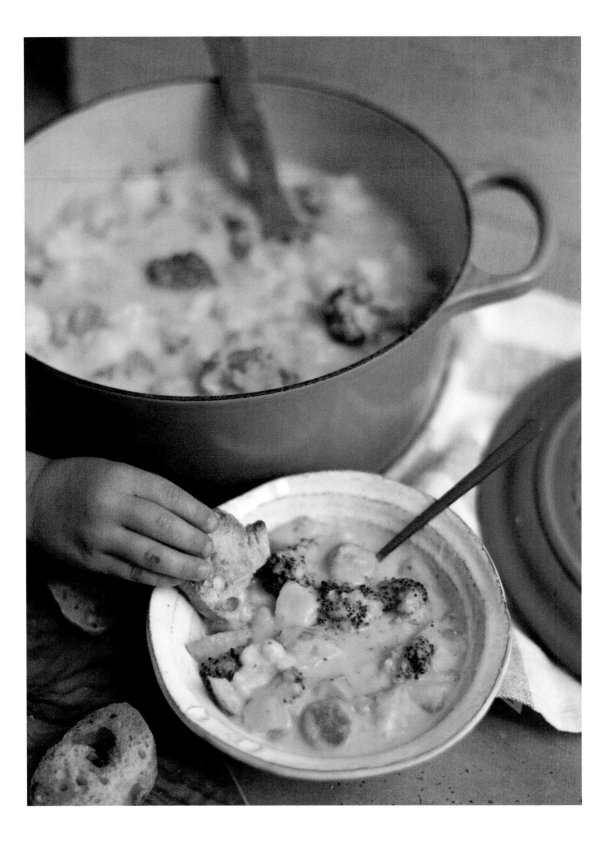

Broccoli Better-Than-Cheddar Soup

This cozy soup has all the creamy richness your heart desires. We love serving it with sourdough bread for dipping or topping it with toasted Ezekiel bread "croutons." Just toast your favorite whole wheat bread and chop into squares!

SERVES 4 TO 6 | TIME: 40 MINUTES

1 yellow onion, diced
3 garlic cloves, minced
2 celery stalks, diced
3 medium carrots, peeled and diced
3 cups vegetable broth or filtered water
6 medium yellow potatoes, cubed
1 head broccoli, cut into small florets
1 head cauliflower, cut into small florets

2 cups plain, unsweetened plant milk
½ cup nutritional yeast
½ cup raw cashews, soaked for at least 30 minutes or ideally 3 to 4 hours and drained (optional, but they make the soup creamy, richer, and more indulgent)
Sea salt and freshly ground black pepper to taste
Lemon wedges, for garnish

1. In a large pot over medium heat, sauté the onion and garlic in a splash of water. When they are translucent, add the celery and carrots and continue cooking until they are soft.
2. Add the vegetable broth and potatoes and bring to a boil over medium-high heat.
3. In a steamer basket over a medium pot filled with 1 inch of water over high heat, steam the broccoli and cauliflower until fork-tender.
4. Add the broccoli, cauliflower, and plant milk to the pot and mix well.
5. To a high-speed blender, add two cups of the soup, the nutritional yeast, and the cashews (if using). Blend until smooth and add back into the pot, stirring to combine.
6. Season with salt and pepper and serve with lemon wedges. A squeeze of lemon amps up the flavor! Leftovers keep best in an airtight container in the refrigerator for up to 3 days.

Butternut Squash Bisque & Two-Ingredient Flatbread

There's nothing more soothing and grounding than a warm bowl of bisque on a chilly evening, especially with tasty flatbread to use for dipping. Try subbing the butternut squash for another bisque-friendly ingredient such as sweet potato, carrot, or tomato, to change the flavor. This two-ingredient gluten-free flatbread is so easy to make it is sure to quickly become a staple in your household!

SERVES 4 | TIME: 30 MINUTES

Butternut Squash Bisque

4 cups vegetable broth or filtered water, plus more as needed

1 butternut squash or other squash, peeled, gutted, and cubed

3 medium carrots, peeled and sliced

1 sweet yellow onion, diced

3 garlic cloves, minced

2 teaspoons freshly grated ginger (optional)

2 teaspoons freshly grated turmeric (optional)

2 teaspoons curry powder (optional)

Dash of cayenne pepper (optional)

Sea salt and freshly ground black pepper to taste

¼ cup unsweetened coconut milk (optional, for a rich, creamy consistency and added flavor)

Sprinkle of pumpkin seeds, for garnish

Dried parsley, for garnish

1. In a large pot over high heat, bring the vegetable broth to a boil. Add the squash and carrots and reduce to medium heat.
2. In a medium frying pan, add a splash of vegetable broth and sauté the onion and garlic on medium-low heat until translucent. Add the ginger, turmeric, curry powder, and cayenne pepper (if using), as well as the salt and pepper and stir for about 30 seconds, or until fragrant.
3. Add the onion mixture to the pot and continue to cook on medium-low until the squash and carrots are cooked through and fork-tender.
4. Add the soup to a high-speed blender and blend until smooth. Return to the pot, stir in the coconut milk, and warm over medium-low heat until ready to serve. Dish up into bowls and sprinkle with pumpkin seeds and dried parsley.

Two-Ingredient Flatbread

1 cup rolled oats or dried red lentils

Coconut oil, for the pan

Suggested spices/garnishes: sea salt, freshly ground black pepper, curry powder, nutritional yeast, dried parsley, maple syrup, and/or coconut sugar (optional)

1. In a high-speed blender, blend oats and 1 cup filtered water until smooth. Allow to sit for 5 minutes.
2. Use a paper towel to add a very thin layer of coconut oil to a frying pan. Place the pan over medium heat.
3. When the pan is hot, pour half the batter into the frying pan and cook for 1 to 2 minutes, or until the edges are slightly brown. Flip and cook the other side for an additional 1 to 2 minutes.
4. Serve alongside the bisque. Leftovers keep best in an airtight container in the refrigerator for up to 3 days.

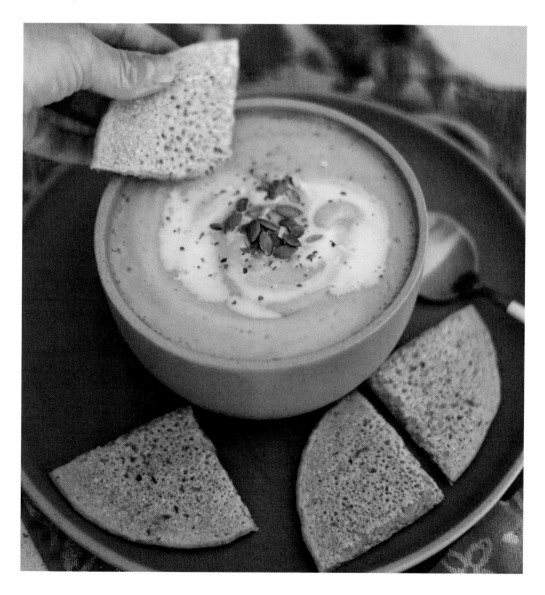

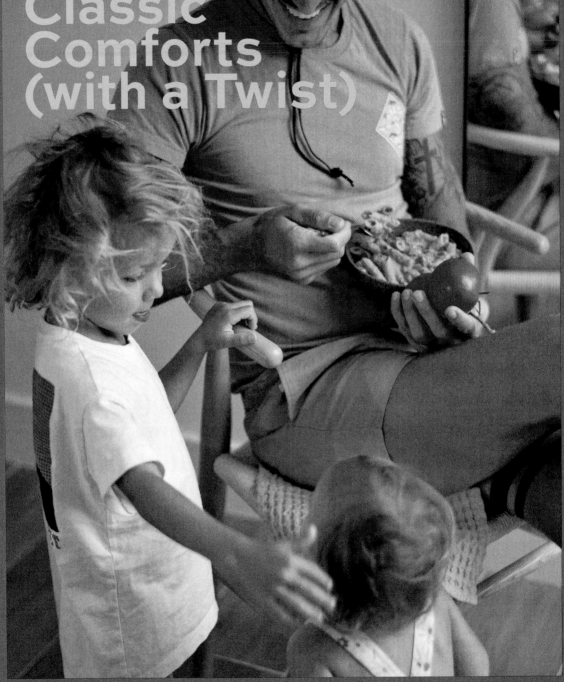

Classic
Comforts
(with a Twist)

If you're looking to wow your guests, this is the section for you! These recipes are familiar classics that we've put our own health-ified, flavor-packed twist on. A family favorite around here is the Garden Greens Lasagna (page 173) that's got more protein and iron and less fat than traditional lasagna, without sacrificing on flavor. Have fun with your own "taco bar" using our Tasty Lentil Quinoa Tacos recipe (page 170)!

Tasty Lentil Quinoa Tacos

With a meaty texture and packed with a complete protein and iron, this lentil quinoa taco "meat" is the perfect filling to please any palate. This fiesta deserves all the fixins!

SERVES 4 TO 6 | TIME: 30 MINUTES

1 cup quinoa, rinsed

1 cup dried green lentils, rinsed

½ red onion, diced

3 garlic cloves, minced

¼ cup walnut pieces (optional)

4 tablespoons nutritional yeast

1 tablespoon dried oregano

1 tablespoon ground cumin

1 tablespoon chili powder

1 tablespoon garlic powder

Sea salt and freshly ground black pepper to taste

4 to 6 soft or hard taco shells

Shredded lettuce, diced tomatoes, diced peppers, Grateful Green Guacamole (page 215), Perfect Pico de Gallo (page 218), Creamy Cashew Cheeze (page 219), and/or lime wedges, for topping

1. In a large pot over medium-high heat, bring 2 cups filtered water to a boil and add the quinoa. Reduce the heat to medium and allow to cook for 10 to 15 minutes or until the water is absorbed. Fluff the quinoa with a fork and remove from the heat.

2. In a separate large pot over medium-high heat, bring 2 cups filtered water to a boil and add the lentils. Reduce the heat to medium and allow the lentils to cook for 10 to 15 minutes or until the water is absorbed and the lentils are soft.

3. While the quinoa and lentils are cooking, sauté the onion and garlic in a medium frying pan with a splash of water until they are translucent.

4. Rinse the cooked lentils under cold water, place in a food processor with the walnuts (if using), and pulse to achieve a "meaty" texture.

5. In a large bowl, combine the lentils, quinoa, onion, garlic, nutritional yeast, oregano, cumin, chili powder, garlic powder, salt, and pepper.

6. Serve in soft or hard taco shells and load them up with your desired toppings and garnishes. Leftovers keep best in individual airtight containers in the refrigerator for up to 3 days.

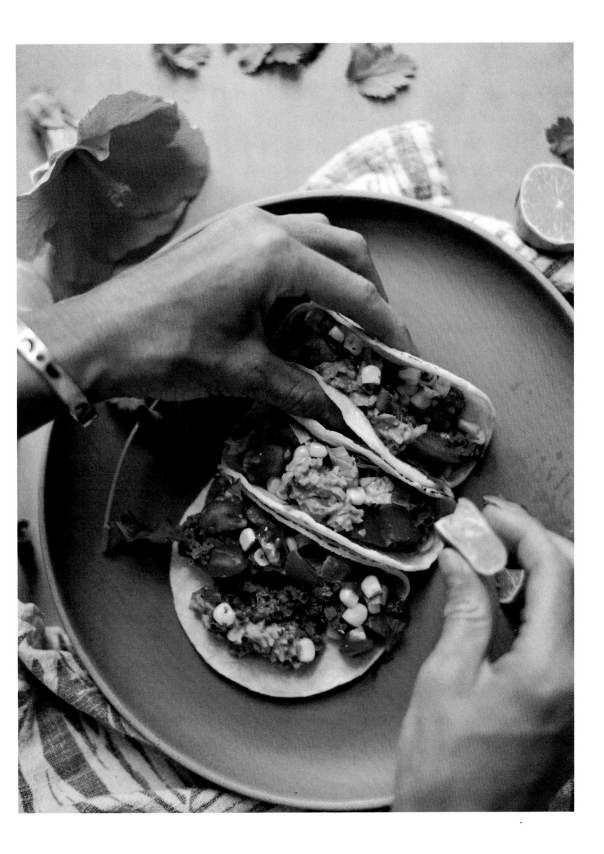

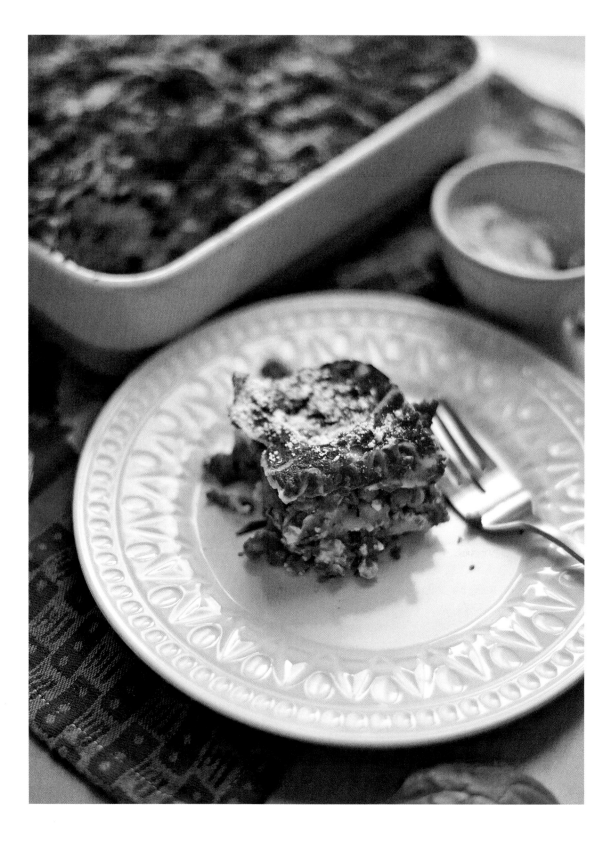

Garden Greens Lasagna with Cashew Parmesan

This lasagna is so easy to make and tastes just like the original classic you know and love. The best part is it's high in protein and flavor and lower in fat than typical dairy-based versions.

SERVES 6 TO 8 | TIME: 75 MINUTES

1 box gluten-free lasagna noodles, cooked according to package directions

2 heaping cups fresh spinach leaves

Lentil Marinara Sauce
1 cup dried green lentils

2 (28-ounce) cans tomato puree

Tofu Ricotta
1 (14-ounce) block extra-firm tofu or Red Lentil Tofu (page 117)
½ cup nutritional yeast
Juice of 1 lemon (2 to 3 tablespoons)

1 teaspoon sea salt
1 teaspoon dried oregano
1 teaspoon dried basil
1 teaspoon garlic powder

Cashew Parmesan
¼ cup raw cashews
1 teaspoon sea salt

2 tablespoons nutritional yeast

1. Preheat the oven to 375°F.
2. To make the sauce, in a large pot over medium-high heat, bring 2 cups filtered water to a boil and add the lentils. Reduce the heat to medium and allow to cook for 10 to 15 minutes or until the water is absorbed and the lentils are soft. Add the tomato puree, mix, and set aside.
3. To make the tofu ricotta, in a large bowl, crumble the tofu until it resembles ricotta. Add the nutritional yeast, lemon juice, salt, oregano, basil, and garlic powder and mix well with a fork.
4. Spread 1 cup of sauce over the bottom of a 9 × 13-inch baking dish.
5. Top with a single layer of lasagna noodles, followed by a layer of tofu ricotta and a layer of spinach. Repeat with another layer of sauce, noodles, ricotta, and spinach. Add another layer as follows: sauce, noodles, ricotta, spinach, sauce, noodles. Top with the rest of the sauce, cover with aluminum foil, and bake in the oven for 40 minutes.
6. Remove the aluminum foil and bake uncovered for 15 minutes.
7. Remove from the oven and let sit for 15 minutes before serving.
8. To make the cashew parmesan, add the cashews, salt, and nutritional yeast to a high-speed blender and blend until the mixture resembles parmesan cheese.
9. Serve slices of lasagna with a sprinkle of cashew parmesan on top and more on the side. Leftovers keep best in an airtight container in the refrigerator for up to 3 days.

Spaghetti & Meat(less) Balls

Spaghetti is always a crowd-pleaser and our low-fat meat(less) lentil balls are so flavorful and juicy that even nonplant-based eaters will be won over!

SERVES 4 TO 5 | TIME: 40 MINUTES

Spaghetti and Tomato Sauce

1 (12-ounce) box brown rice, chickpea, or lentil spaghetti noodles

¼ cup vegetable broth or filtered water

3 to 4 garlic cloves, minced

1 sweet yellow onion, diced

1 (14.5-ounce) can diced tomatoes

1 cup tomato puree (optional, for a less chunky, more soupy sauce)

2 tablespoons tomato paste

1 tablespoon dried basil

1 tablespoon dried oregano

Sea salt and freshly ground black pepper to taste

Meat(less) Balls

3 garlic cloves, minced

½ small yellow onion, diced

1½ cups cooked green lentils

¾ cup chickpea flour

5 tablespoons nutritional yeast

1 tablespoon tomato paste

1 tablespoon flaxseeds

1½ tablespoons Italian seasoning

1 teaspoon dried parsley

Sea salt and freshly ground black pepper to taste

Cashew Parmesan (page 173) and fresh basil leaves, for garnish

1. Preheat the oven to 350°F. Line a baking sheet with parchment paper.
2. Cook the noodles according to the package directions and set aside.
3. To make the sauce, in a large sauté pan over medium heat, add the broth and sauté the garlic and onion until translucent. Add the diced tomatoes, tomato puree (if using), and tomato paste, basil, oregano, salt, and pepper. Reduce the heat to medium-low, and cook for 10 minutes stirring often.
4. To make the meat(less) balls, in a large sauté pan over medium heat, sauté the garlic and onion in a splash of water until translucent. Add the garlic, onion, lentils, flour, nutritional yeast, tomato paste, flaxseeds, Italian seasoning, parsley, salt, and pepper to a food processor and pulse until the consistency is even and clumpy. Form into 2-tablespoon-size balls and bake on the prepared baking sheet for 10 to 15 minutes, or until slightly browned and firm on the outside.
5. Portion the spaghetti into bowls and top with sauce and meat(less) balls. Garnish with a dusting of Cashew Parmesan and fresh basil. Leftovers keep best in an airtight container in the refrigerator for up to 3 days.

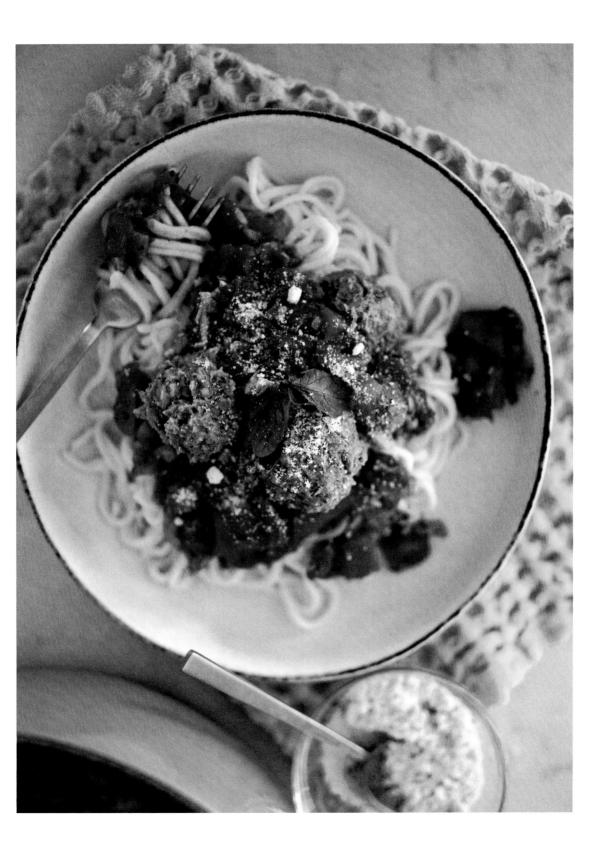

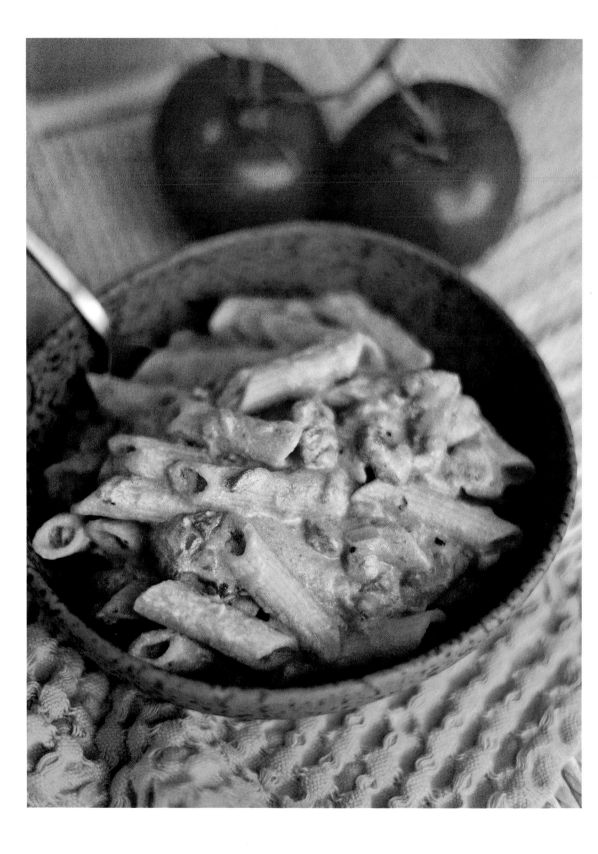

Creamy One-Pot Vodka(less) Penne Pasta

This is a rich and indulgent pasta recipe that also happens to be low in fat and high in protein. We always make this guilt-free favorite for family and friends and it's a hit among vegans and nonvegans alike!

SERVES 6 | TIME: 30 MINUTES

2 cups vegetable broth
1 small sweet onion, diced
3 garlic cloves, minced
1 teaspoon oregano
Sea salt and freshly ground black pepper to taste
2 cups fresh or canned diced tomatoes
1 tablespoon tomato paste

2 cups unsweetened plant milk (we like organic soy)
2 (16-ounce) boxes gluten-free pasta (we like brown rice, chickpea, or lentil)
Red pepper flakes to taste (optional)
Cashew Parmesan (page 173), for garnish

1. In a large pot over medium-high heat, add 1 to 2 tablespoons of the vegetable broth and sauté the onion, garlic, oregano, salt, and pepper until the onion is translucent.
2. Add the diced tomatoes and tomato paste and continue to cook for 5 minutes.
3. Add the remaining vegetable broth, plant milk, and pasta and cook on medium-low for 15 minutes or until the sauce thickens, stirring continually so the pasta doesn't stick to the bottom.
4. Remove from the heat and serve topped with red pepper flakes (if using) and our super easy Cashew Parmesan. Leftovers keep best in an airtight container in the refrigerator for up to 3 days.

(Un)boxed Mac & Cheeze Powder

This vegan mac and cheeze powder is super easy to prep and makes quick meals a breeze. Just keep the powder in the refrigerator and grab it in a pinch! Plus it's so much healthier than store-bought.

MAKES 1½ CUPS POWDER | TIME: 20 MINUTES

½ cup raw cashews
½ cup nutritional yeast
3 tablespoons oat flour
2 tablespoons arrowroot starch or other starch
1½ teaspoons sea salt
2 teaspoons garlic powder
2 teaspoons onion powder

2 teaspoons paprika
1 teaspoon mustard powder
Crack of freshly ground black pepper
Dash of ground turmeric
1 (12-ounce) box gluten-free pasta, for serving
1 cup unsweetened plant milk, for serving

1. Add the cashews, nutritional yeast, flour, arrowroot, salt, garlic powder, onion powder, paprika, mustard powder, black pepper, and turmeric to a high-speed blender and blend until a well-combined powder forms. Store in a mason jar in a cool, dark pantry for up to a month or longer in the refrigerator.

When you are ready to make mac and cheeze:

2. Cook the pasta according to the package directions. Drain, rinse, and return the pasta to the pot.
3. Place ⅓ to ½ cup mac and cheeze powder and plant milk into a high-speed blender and blend until smooth. Start with less powder and add more to achieve desired level of flavor.
4. Pour the sauce over the pasta, mix, and warm over low heat until the sauce becomes creamy and thick. Best served with a glass of your favorite plant milk.

Notes: To make nut-free: Replace the cashews with the same amount of seeds such as pumpkin, hemp, or sunflower.

To make no-/low-fat: Replace the cashews with same amount of oat flour.

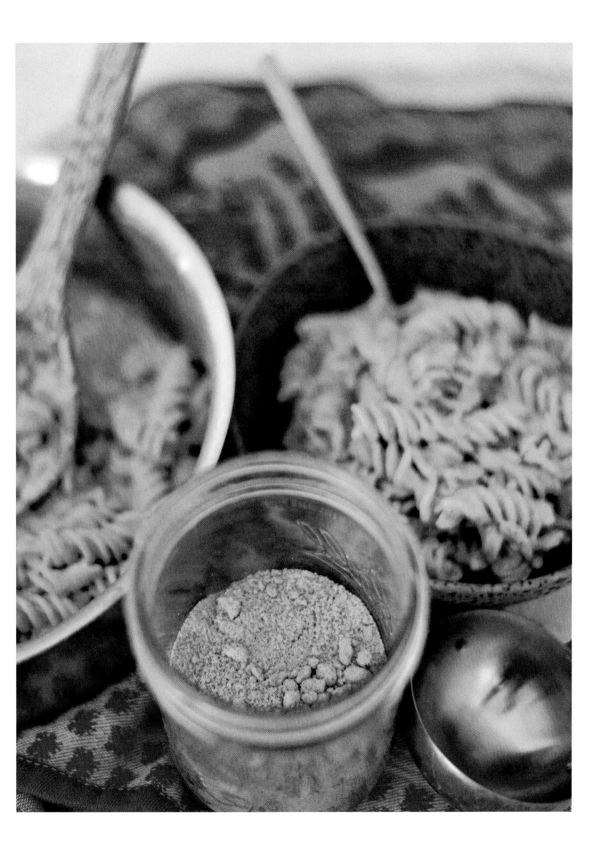

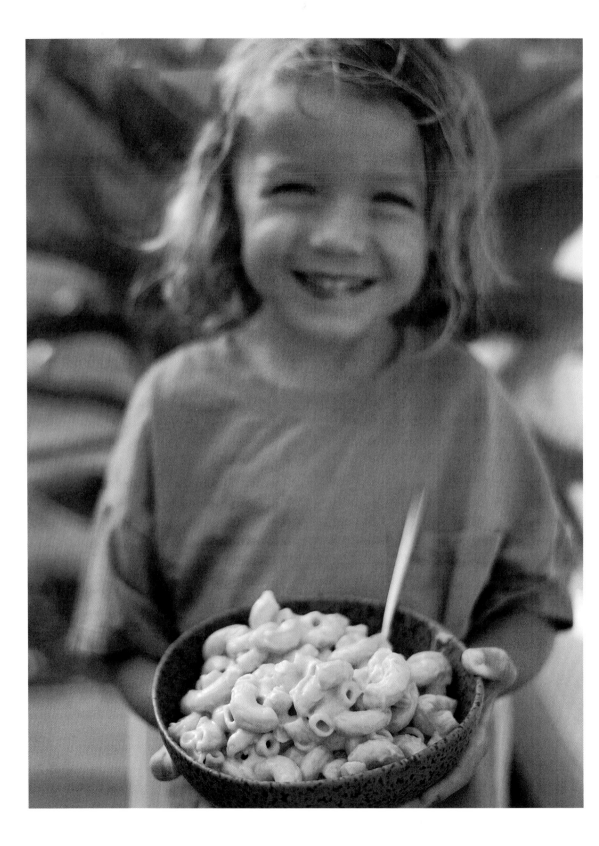

Creamy Veggie Mac & Cheeze

The plant-based version of this childhood favorite is pure magic! It's ripe with hidden veggies and has all the creamy goodness you remember.

(K) | SERVES 6 | TIME: 30 MINUTES

2 (15-ounce) boxes chickpea elbow pasta
1 large Yukon Gold potato, peeled and boiled
4 medium carrots, peeled and boiled
3 garlic cloves, boiled
1 red bell pepper, chopped
½ cup raw cashews, soaked for 3 to 4 hours and drained (add more for a creamier dish!)

½ cup nutritional yeast
½ teaspoon turmeric (for color)
1 teaspoon sea salt
Smoked paprika to taste (optional)
Cayenne pepper or red pepper flakes to taste (optional)
Juice of 1 lemon

1. Cook the pasta according to the package directions and set aside.
2. Add the potato, carrots, garlic, bell pepper, cashews, nutritional yeast, turmeric, salt, paprika (if using), cayenne pepper (if using), lemon juice, and ½ cup filtered water to a high-speed blender and blend until smooth and creamy.
3. In a large bowl, mix the cheeze sauce into the pasta and enjoy! Leftovers keep best in an airtight container in the refrigerator for up to 3 days.

Notes: For an extra-festive fall twist, replace the potato and carrots with 3 cups cubed butternut squash or pumpkin.

For a nut-free and lower-fat dish: Omit the cashews or use ½ cup sunflower seeds instead.

Shepherd's Veggie Pot Pie

This is the epitome of healthy comfort food. It checks all the boxes: tons of veggies, plenty of protein, and a hearty and delicious taste!

SERVES 4 TO 6 | TIME: 40 MINUTES

2 cups vegetable broth, plus more as needed

1 cup dried green or brown lentils, rinsed

8 medium Yukon Gold potatoes, peeled and chopped

¼ cup nutritional yeast, plus more to taste (see Step 3)

Sea salt and freshly ground black pepper to taste

2 cups unsweetened plant milk, plus more as needed

1 yellow onion, diced

3 or 4 garlic cloves, minced

3 medium carrots, peeled and diced

1 head broccoli, cut into small florets

½ cup baby bella mushrooms, finely chopped

1 cup frozen sweet corn

1 cup frozen peas

2 tablespoons arrowroot starch

Chopped fresh parsley, for garnish

1. Preheat the oven to 375°F.
2. In a large pot over high heat, bring the vegetable broth to a boil. Add the lentils, reduce the heat to medium, and cook until the water is absorbed. Set aside.
3. In a large pot over high heat, cover the potatoes in water and boil until fork-tender. Drain the water. Mash to your liking and season with nutritional yeast, salt, and pepper to taste. Add a splash of plant milk to make it creamier, if desired.
4. In a large pot over medium heat, sauté the onion, garlic, and carrots in a splash of vegetable broth until tender, about 7 minutes. Add the broccoli, mushrooms, corn, and peas and sauté for a few minutes or until the broccoli is bright green and tender.
5. Add the 2 cups of plant milk, ¼ cup nutritional yeast, arrowroot, salt, pepper, and lentils, stir to combine and cook over medium-low heat until the liquid thickens, about 7 minutes.
6. To a 9 × 13-inch baking dish, add the veggie-lentil blend and top with a spread of mashed potatoes. Bake for 15 minutes. Bake under the broiler for 2 to 3 minutes more, or until the top is slightly golden.
7. Remove from the oven and allow to cool for 5 minutes before serving. Garnish with a dusting of parsley and dig in! Leftovers keep best in an airtight container in the refrigerator for up to 3 days.

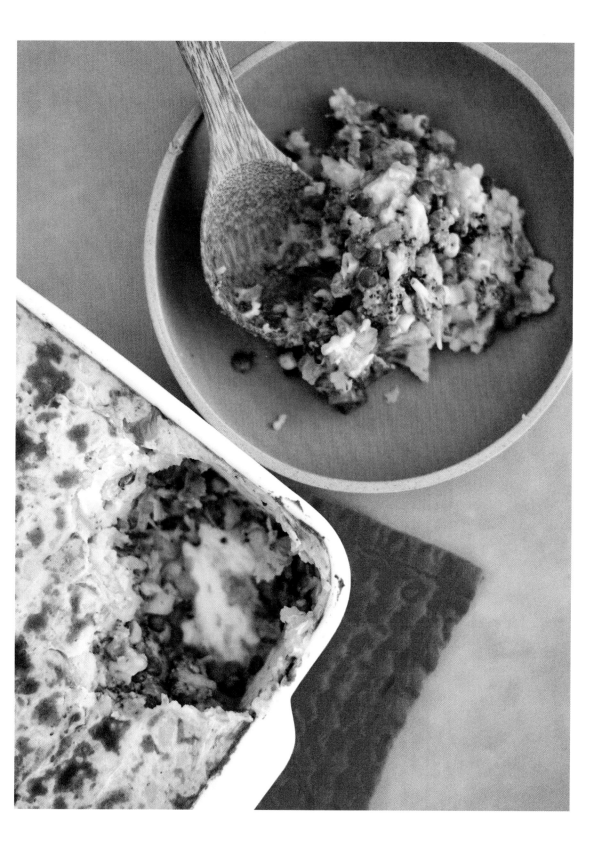

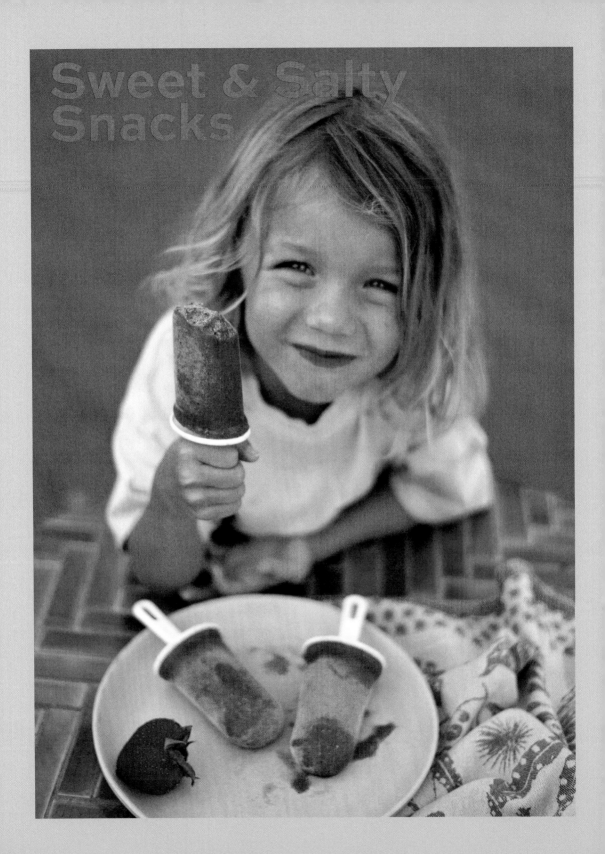

Sweet & Salty
Snacks

Snacking isn't a bad thing—we just need to snack with purpose and intention! Whether you're in the mood for something sweet, salty, chewy, or crunchy, we've got you covered. The key is to make at least one of these recipes each week to have on hand to keep less healthy cravings at bay. We love to bake up a batch of Strawberry Banana Muffins (page 191) or Superfood Brownies (page 188) to bring with us or grab for a midday snack.

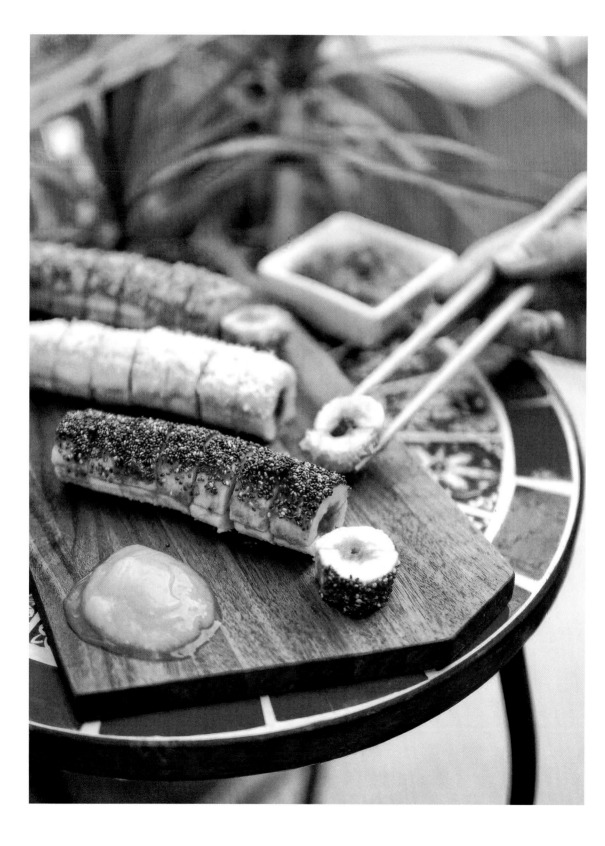

Banana Sushi

Have fun with fruit! Sometimes simply changing up the presentation can make a world of difference, especially when it comes to feeding littles. Try different fillings and/or toppings to keep things interesting—and sneak in some extra nutrition.

(R) | SERVES 1 | TIME: 5 MINUTES

1 ripe banana
2 tablespoons nut butter of choice

Date Paste
8 to 10 Medjool dates, pitted
Hemp seeds, chia seeds, coconut flakes, cacao powder, and/or ground cinnamon, for topping (optional)

Fruit Puree
1 cup frozen raspberries, thawed
1 tablespoon maple syrup

1. Peel the banana and slice it down the middle. Carefully scrape out a little bit of the middle from each banana half, creating a shallow well.
2. To make the date paste, soak the dates in warm water for 20 minutes. Add them to a high-speed blender with just enough soaking water to cover and blend until smooth.
3. To make the fruit puree, add the raspberries and maple syrup to a mini blender and blend until smooth.
4. Into each banana well, spread 1 tablespoon of nut butter and 1 tablespoon of date paste. Put the two halves back together and spread the remaining nut butter and date paste on top.
5. Sprinkle with hemp seeds, coconut flakes, or other desired toppings. Slice into bite-size pieces and serve with fruit puree for dipping.

Notes: Pop leftovers into the freezer for delicious bite-size treats!
Store extra date paste and fruit puree in airtight containers in the refrigerator for 4 to 5 days.

Superfood Brownies

These delicious, gluten-free, and refined-sugar-free brownies are the best guilt-free fuel to enjoy any time of day! They were also one of my favorite treats while I was breastfeeding because they contain a handful of ingredients found to boost milk supply, such as oats, flaxseeds, chia seeds, dates, and cacao. Worked for me! That being said, they're also kid- and Dad-friendly, too!

MAKES 16 | TIME: 60 MINUTES

15 Medjool dates, pitted
2 ripe bananas
2 cups rolled oats
4 tablespoons ground chia seeds or flaxseeds
4 tablespoons cacao powder
1 teaspoon vanilla bean powder or extract
1 teaspoon ground cinnamon
1 tablespoon baking powder

½ teaspoon baking soda
½ teaspoon sea salt
1 scoop chocolate plant-based protein powder (optional)
2 tablespoons brewer's yeast (optional, but may help increase milk supply)
Creamy Vanilla Plant Milk (page 75), for serving

1. Preheat the oven to 350°F.
2. In a medium bowl, add the pitted dates, cover with warm water, and soak for 20 minutes. Place the soaked dates, half of their soaking water, and the bananas into a high-speed blender and blend into a smooth paste. Set aside.
3. Place the rolled oats and chia seeds in a high-speed blender and blend to a fine flour.
4. In a large bowl, combine the oat flour, cacao powder, vanilla, cinnamon, baking powder, baking soda, salt, protein powder, and brewer's yeast (if using).
5. Add the date paste to the oat mixture and mix until well combined.
6. Pour the batter into a 9 × 13-inch baking dish lined with parchment and bake for 30 to 35 minutes, or until a toothpick inserted into the middle comes out clean. Remove from the oven and allow to cool for 10 minutes. Enjoy with a glass of Creamy Vanilla Plant Milk. Store the brownies in an airtight container in the refrigerator for up to 5 days.

Note: If you prefer, replace the protein powder and/or brewer's yeast with ½ cup rolled oats.

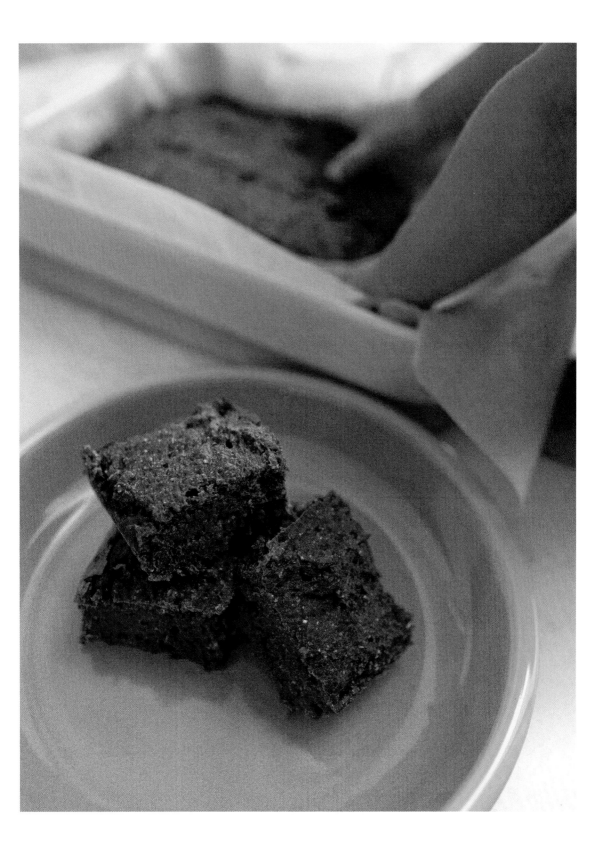

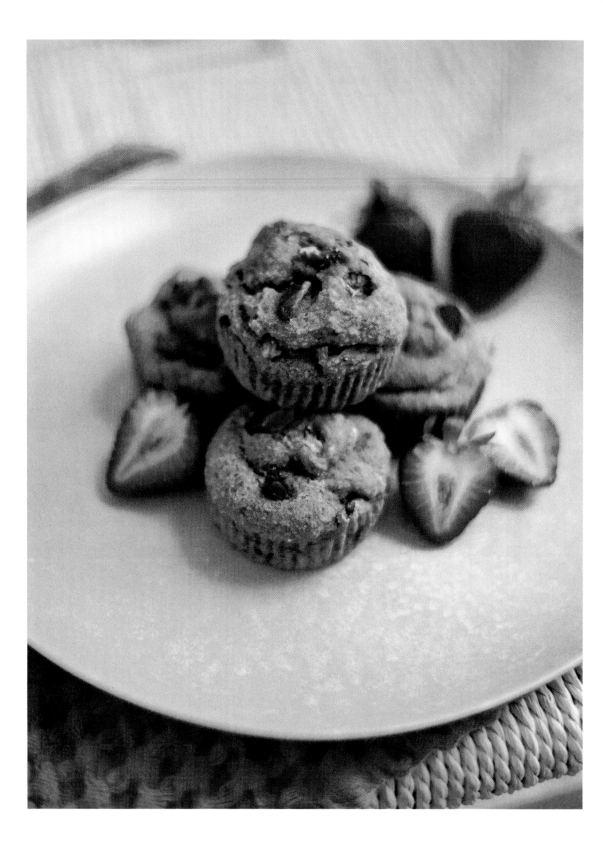

Strawberry Banana Muffins

Max and Liv love these sweet treats, and so do we! They're ripe with healthy carbs, omega-3s, iron, and protein.

(K) | MAKES 12 MUFFINS | TIME: 40 MINUTES

15 Medjool dates, pitted

2 ripe bananas

4 tablespoons raw tahini or nut
or seed butter of choice

1 teaspoon apple cider vinegar

3½ cups rolled oats

2 tablespoons ground chia seeds or flaxseeds

1 tablespoon baking powder

½ teaspoon baking soda

1 teaspoon vanilla bean powder or extract

1 teaspoon ground cinnamon

½ teaspoon sea salt

1 scoop vanilla plant-based
protein powder (optional)

Splash of unsweetened plant milk, or to taste

6 large strawberries, diced

Creamy Vanilla Plant Milk (page 75), for serving

1. Preheat the oven to 350°F.
2. In a medium bowl, add the pitted dates, cover with warm water, and soak for 20 minutes. Place the soaked dates, half of their soaking water, the bananas, tahini, and apple cider vinegar into a high-speed blender and blend into a smooth paste. Set aside.
3. Place the rolled oats and chia seeds in a high-speed blender and blend to a fine flour.
4. In a large mixing bowl, combine the oat flour, baking powder, baking soda, vanilla, cinnamon, salt, and protein powder (if using).
5. Add the date paste to the oat mixture and mix until well combined. Mix in a splash of plant milk if the batter is too dry and the flour isn't thoroughly mixed in. Mix in the strawberries.
6. Pour the batter into a muffin tray lined with parchment-paper baking cups and bake for 25 to 30 minutes, or until golden on top and a toothpick inserted into the middle comes out clean. Remove from the oven and allow to cool for 10 minutes. Enjoy with a glass of Creamy Vanilla Plant Milk. Store the muffins in an airtight container in the refrigerator for up to 5 days.

Note: Switch things up and replace the strawberries with 1 cup blueberries, raspberries, diced pineapple, or chopped bananas.

Savory Veggie Muffins

These muffins are a sneaky way to turn a veggie skeptic into a veggie lover! They're a super nutritious baby- and kid-friendly savory snack. Try these dunked in our Quinoa Veggie Immunity Soup (page 151).

MAKES 10 MUFFINS | TIME: 40 MINUTES

1 tablespoon flaxseeds
1 tablespoon chia seeds
¾ cup unsweetened plant milk (we like organic soy)
2 cups chickpea flour
3 tablespoons nutritional yeast
1 teaspoon baking powder
1 teaspoon baking soda
1 teaspoon sea salt
Crack of freshly ground black pepper

½ teaspoon dried parsley
½ teaspoon garlic powder
½ teaspoon onion powder
½ medium carrot, grated (about ½ cup)
⅓ medium zucchini, unpeeled and grated (about ½ cup)
¼ red bell pepper, grated (about ½ cup)
1 cup finely chopped fresh spinach leaves
1 teaspoon apple cider vinegar

1. Preheat the oven to 350°F.
2. Place the flaxseeds and chia seeds in a high-speed blender and blend to a fine powder. In a small bowl, combine with the plant milk and set aside to thicken.
3. In a large mixing bowl, add the chickpea flour, nutritional yeast, baking powder, baking soda, salt, pepper, parsley, garlic powder, and onion powder and mix well to combine.
4. In a separate large mixing bowl, combine the carrot, zucchini, pepper, and spinach.
5. Add ½ cup filtered water and the veggies, flaxseed mixture, and apple cider vinegar to the dry ingredients and mix well.
6. Pour the batter into a muffin tray lined with parchment-paper baking cups and bake for about 20 minutes, or until golden brown on top and a toothpick poked into the middle comes out clean. Remove from the oven and allow to cool for 10 minutes before eating. Store the muffins in an airtight container in the refrigerator for up to 5 days.

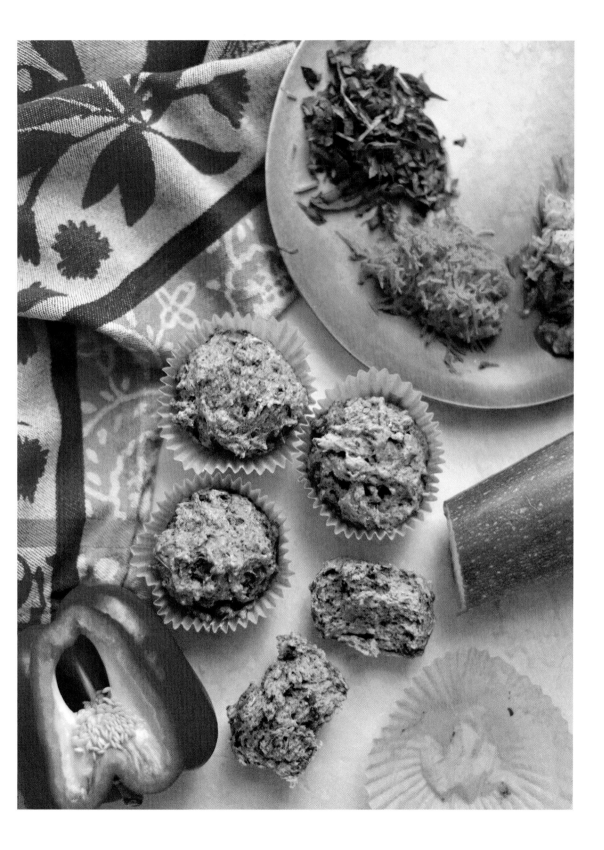

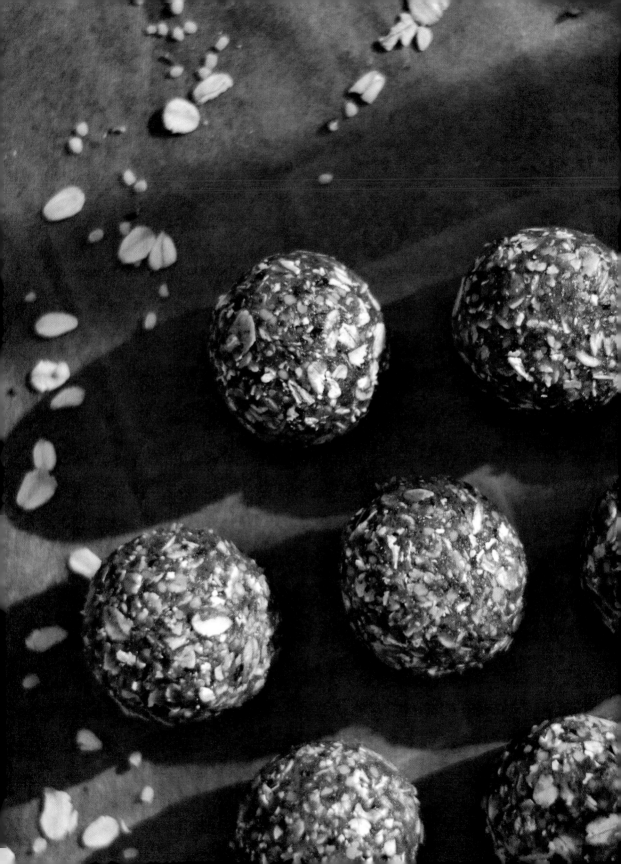

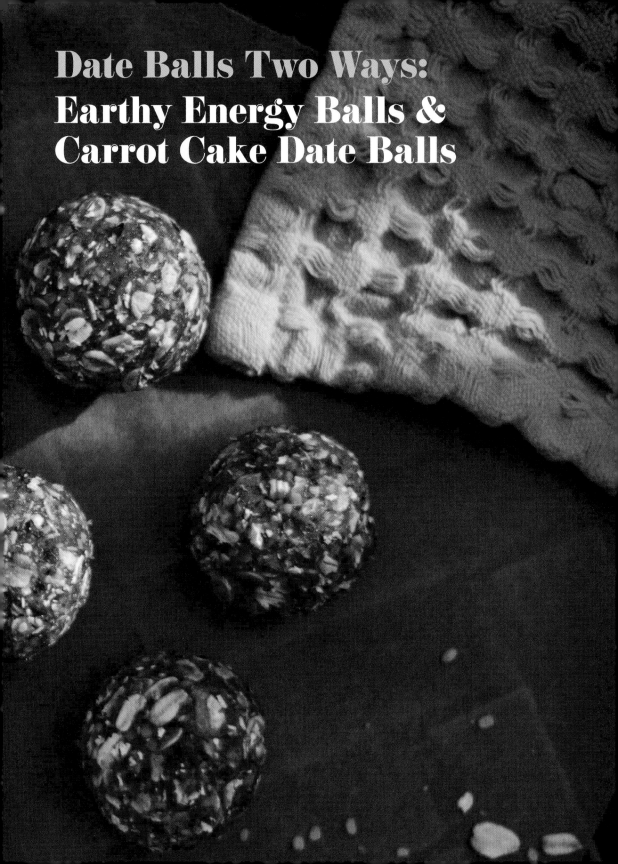

Date Balls Two Ways:
Earthy Energy Balls &
Carrot Cake Date Balls

Earthy Energy Balls

An easy snack to grab 'n' go on the way to sporting events, they're super energizing, thanks to the concentrated dose of healthy carbs and fats.

(R) | MAKES 10 TO 12 BALLS | TIME: 20 MINUTES

15 Medjool dates, pitted
¼ cup almond or peanut butter
1 tablespoon maple syrup
1 teaspoon vanilla bean powder or extract

Pinch of sea salt
1 cup rolled oats
2 tablespoons hemp seeds
1 teaspoon ground cinnamon

1. In a medium bowl, add the pitted dates, cover with warm water, and soak for 20 minutes.
2. Place the dates, nut butter, maple syrup, vanilla, and salt into a food processor and process until a large ball forms.
3. In a large bowl, add the oats, hemp, and cinnamon and mix well.
4. Add the date ball to the bowl and mash and mix until all the ingredients are well combined.
5. Using your hands, roll 1 tablespoon of the mixture into a ball and place on a baking sheet. Repeat until all the mixture has been used. Place them in the refrigerator for at least 30 minutes to firm up, and enjoy!

Note: Try adding ¼ cup cacao or carob powder to the food processor or mixing in dark chocolate chips with the oats for a chocolaty twist.

Carrot Cake Date Balls

These date balls are a real treat with a sneaky veggie included. They're the perfect bite-size version of one of the most classically delicious kinds of cake!

(R) | MAKES 16 TO 20 BALLS | TIME: 10 MINUTES

15 Medjool dates, pitted
2 medium carrots, peeled and chopped
½ cup rolled oats
¼ cup nut butter (we like cashew butter)
2 tablespoons pecans

2 teaspoons hemp seeds
1 teaspoon vanilla bean powder or extract
½ teaspoon ground cinnamon
Pinch of sea salt
3 tablespoons unsweetened shredded coconut

1. In a medium bowl, add the pitted dates, cover with warm water, and soak for 20 minutes.
2. Place the dates, carrots, oats, nut butter, pecans, hemp seeds, vanilla, cinnamon, and salt into a food processor and pulse until a large, gooey ball forms. Add a splash of water if needed to reach the desired consistency. Using your hands, roll 1 tablespoon of the mixture into a ball, place onto a baking sheet or plate, and repeat until all the mixture has been used.
3. On a small plate, sprinkle the coconut and roll each ball in it until well coated. The balls can keep in an airtight container in the refrigerator for up to 5 days or up to 1 month in the freezer.

DIY
date balls

Homemade date balls are perfect for a party plate, dessert bite, lunchbox addition, energizing preworkout snack, or grab 'n' go fuel! They provide plenty of macronutrient nutrition in a bite-size ball, with dates forming the base as our healthy carbohydrate and nut or seed butter (or the nuts and seeds themselves) for fat and protein. You can even mix in protein powder if you choose!

Carbohydrate Base
Begin with 15-20 pitted Medjool dates as your base.

Try it with:
½ to 1 cup rolled oats (optional)

Healthy Fats
¼ to ½ cup nut or seed butter

Try it with:
1-2 varieties of nuts and/or or seeds (walnut, almond, cashew, pumpkin, sunflower, chia, hemp, flax)

Superfoods & Flavor Enhancers
Add 1 to 2 tablespoons of any dried or powdered superfoods / flavor enhancers (maple syrup, peanut butter powder, cacao, shredded coconut, açaí, vanilla bean, protein powder, cinnamon, dried or freeze-dried fruit).

General Steps
Add all ingredients to a food processor and process until a large, gooey ball forms. (Can also choose to only process dates, nuts/seeds, and butters together and roll in oats, superfoods, and flavor enhancers.) Measure out and roll tablespoon-size balls. Balls keep best in the refrigerator for 1 to 2 weeks or in the freezer for up to 3 weeks.

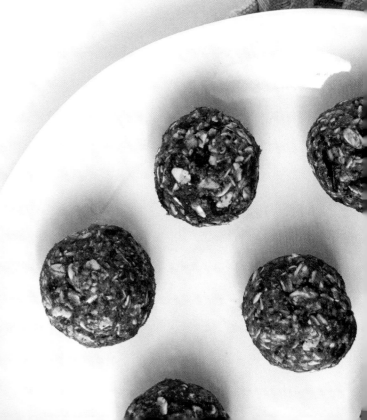

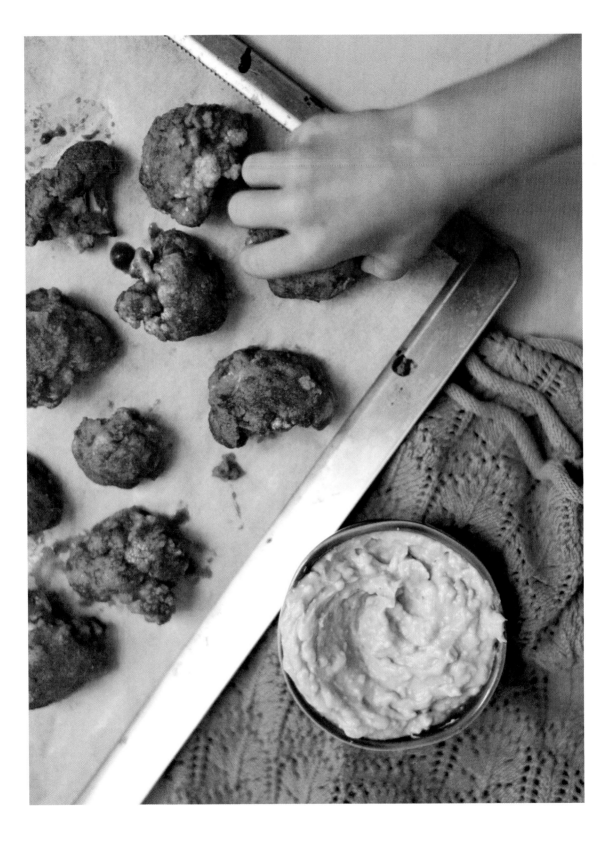

Cauliflower Buffalo Wings

This recipe is a fun and creative way to enjoy one of our favorite and most versatile veggies: cauliflower! Cruciferous veggies like this one are loaded with cancer-fighting compounds, vitamin C, and so much more. This appetizer is the perfect party-pleaser for your favorite sporting event and beyond!

SERVES 2 TO 4 | TIME: 30 MINUTES

1 large head cauliflower, cut into bite-size florets

Grateful Green Guacamole (page 215), for serving

Batter

¾ cup brown rice flour
2 teaspoons onion powder
2 teaspoons garlic powder
1 teaspoon ground cumin

1 teaspoon paprika
¼ teaspoon freshly ground black pepper
¼ teaspoon sea salt

Sauce

1 tablespoon maple syrup
1 tablespoon tamari
1 tablespoon tomato paste
1 tablespoon apple cider vinegar

1 teaspoon garlic powder
1 teaspoon paprika
¼ teaspoon chili powder

1. Preheat the oven to 450°F. Line a baking sheet with parchment paper.
2. To make the batter, in a large bowl, whisk together 1 cup filtered water with the flour, onion powder, garlic powder, cumin, paprika, pepper, and salt.
3. Dunk cauliflower florets into the batter and coat well. Place them on the prepared baking sheet.
4. Bake the florets for 20 minutes, flipping halfway through.
5. To make the sauce, in a bowl, combine 2 tablespoons filtered water with the maple syrup, tamari, tomato paste, vinegar, garlic powder, paprika, and chili powder and mix well. Brush the sauce onto the cooked wings and pop them back into the oven to bake for 3 minutes.
6. Remove from the oven, plate, and serve alongside Grateful Green Guacamole or your favorite dipping sauce.

Easy Cheezy Kale Chips

Craving something crunchy and salty? Look no further than this healthier version of Doritos! Plus, this cheeze sauce is an amazing salad dressing, too.

(R) | SERVES 2 TO 4 | TIME: 55 MINUTES

1 head curly kale, destemmed and torn into bite-size pieces

Cheeze sauce

½ red bell pepper, chopped

1 cup raw cashews, soaked in warm water for four hours or at least 30 minutes, drained and rinsed, or sunflower seeds

1½ tablespoons nutritional yeast

¼ teaspoon sea salt

Juice of ½ lemon

1. Preheat the oven to 300°F. Line a baking sheet with parchment paper. Rinse and dry the kale.
2. To make the sauce, place the bell pepper, cashews, nutritional yeast, salt, and lemon juice into a high-speed blender and blend until smooth.
3. To a large bowl, add the kale and pour the sauce over it, massaging until the leaves are well coated.
4. On the prepared baking sheet, spread the kale chips in an even layer and bake for 25 to 30 minutes, tossing once halfway. Remove them from the oven when the kale chips are crispy but not turning brown or starting to burn. Transfer to a large bowl and crunch away! The chips keep best in an airtight container for up to 5 days.

Note: If you have a dehydrator, spread the kale in an even layer on lined dehydrator trays and dehydrate at 105°F overnight.

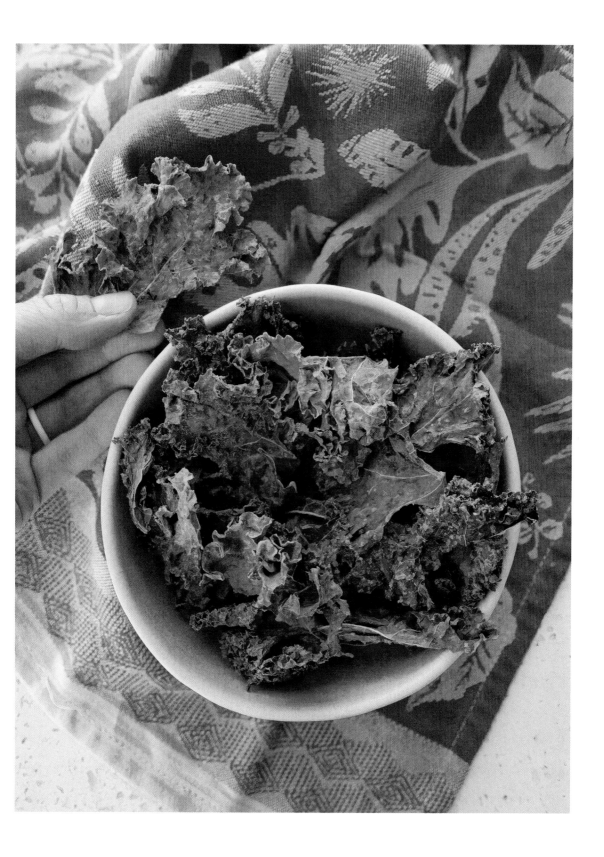

Movie Night Popcorn

Whether you like savory or sweet popcorn (or a mixture of both!), this oil-free, low-calorie, and high-fiber snack is loaded with flavor and makes every movie night special!

MAKES 15 CUPS | TIME: 5 MINUTES

½ cup organic popcorn kernels (yellow or white)
Water in a spray bottle

Savory Seasoning

1 teaspoon sea salt
1 tablespoon nutritional yeast

Sweet Seasoning

1 teaspoon ground cinnamon
1 tablespoon coconut sugar

1. Pop corn kernels in an air popper according the air popper directions. Place in a large bowl and set aside.
2. To make either of the seasonings, add the ingredients to a high-speed blender and blend into a fine powder.
3. Set the spray bottle to fine mist and mist the popcorn from about 1 foot away (not directly onto the popcorn). Immediately dust with seasoning and toss well. Spray again and dust again. Toss and dig in! Keeps best in an airtight container for up to 5 days.

Note: Try combining the salty and sweet seasoning for a kettle corn–inspired flavor.

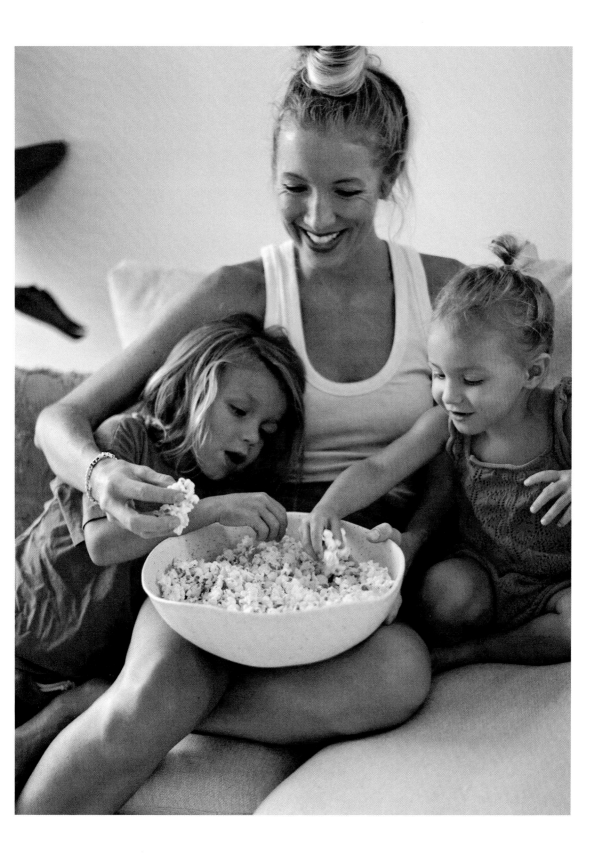

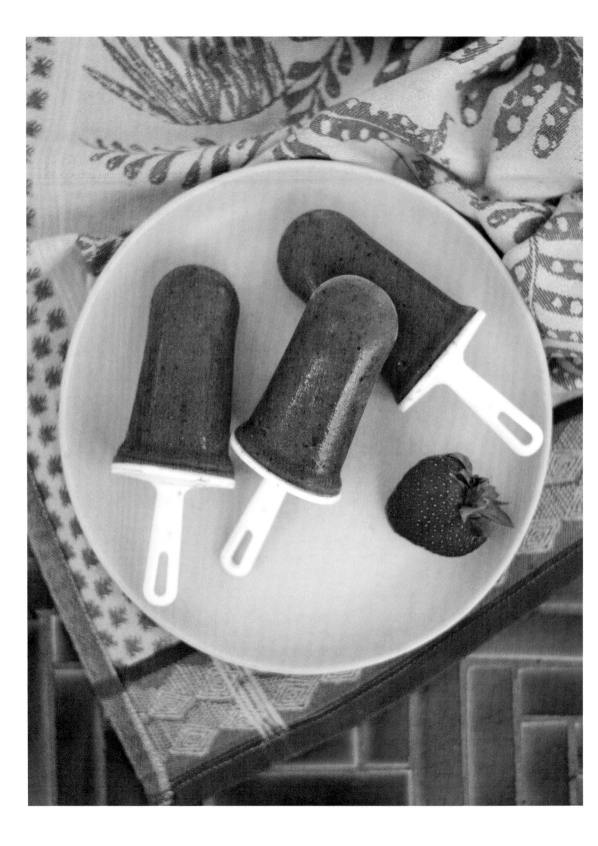

Pink Passion Popsicles

These popsicles are positively perfect: delicious, nutritious, and easy to make. They're loaded with vitamins, antioxidants, electrolytes, and even a little bit of healthy omega-3 fatty acids, thanks to the chia seeds. The best part is—no refined sugar! The secret to making these pink pops irresistible is the tart and tangy taste of passion fruit. Pro tip: anytime you or your little one doesn't finish a smoothie, simply pop the leftovers into a popsicle mold for a refreshing sweet treat!

(R) (K) | SERVES 6 | TIME: 5 MINUTES

1½ frozen ripe bananas

1 cup frozen strawberries

½ frozen pink pitaya pack or
1 tablespoon pitaya powder

½ cup frozen or 3 cups fresh passion fruit

2 cups coconut water

1 tablespoon chia seeds

1 scoop vanilla plant-based
protein powder (optional)

1. Place the bananas, strawberries, pitaya pack, passion fruit, coconut water, chia seeds, and protein powder (if using) in a high-speed blender and blend until smooth.
2. Pour the mixture into popsicle molds and pop in the freezer for 2 hours, or until solid. Remove and find a spot in the sun to enjoy! Popsicles keep in the freezer for up to 1 month.

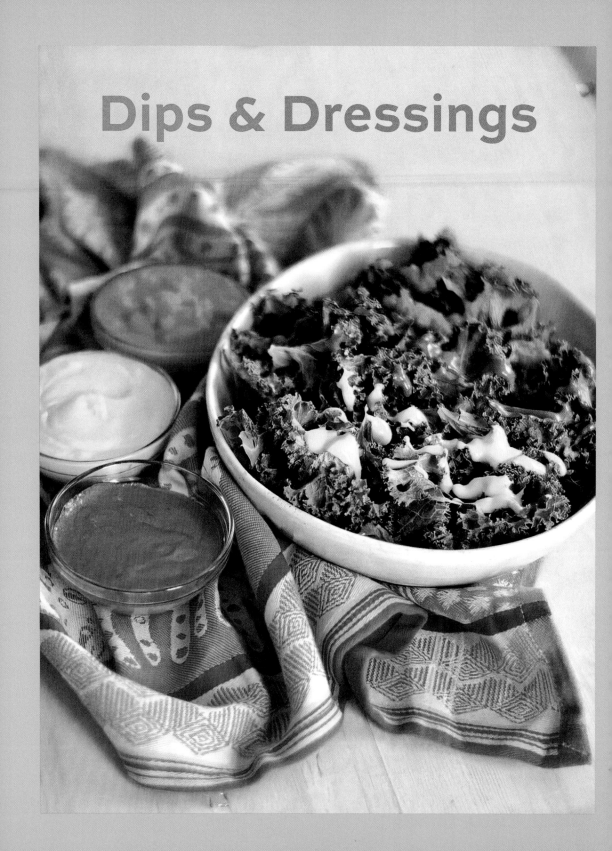

Dips & Dressings

uch like herbs and spices, dips and dressings can take an otherwise bland and boring dish to bold and flavorful. There's something for every meal in here, whether you need to dip, spread, or drizzle to enhance your dishes. Not to mention, adding a dressing with a healthy fat to your salad, for example, will help your body to absorb the maximum amount of nutrition!

un-
dressings

Dressings that aren't really dressings! All it really takes is a healthy fat, which could be a nut, seed, or avocado with the right liquid, like citrus, syrup, aminos, or even just water. You can also get creative with the addition of fruits, veggies, and various seasonings for added flavor and nutrition. Not every dressing needs to contain ingredients from every category, but this is a great place to start!

General guidelines for a serving size of 2 to 4:

Healthy Fats
(¼ cup)

Nuts or seeds: hemp, chia, flax, sunflower, pumpkin, cashews

Nut or seed butters: tahini, peanut, almond, cashew

Other: avocado, coconut meat or milk

Liquid
(2-4 tbsp.)

Citrus: lemon, lime, orange

Sweet: coconut aminos, maple syrup, agave

Savory: tamari, liquid aminos

Other: water, coconut water

Produce
(½ cup chopped)

Fruits: pineapple, mango

Veggies: bell pepper, carrot, zucchini, greens, ginger, sun-dried tomato, garlic

Seasonings
(to taste)

Liquids: miso, apple cider vinegar

Solids: nutritional yeast, salt, pepper, basil, cilantro, curry powder, cumin

Add-ons!
Nutritional yeast (B vitamins, protein, iron, and cheezy flavor), dulse (iodine and other minerals)

Our favorites for salads & balance bowls
(page 119)

Lemon + tahini (tangy + "salty")

Avocado + coconut aminos (sweet + savory)

Make It Your Own

Now let's get a bit more involved and creative! Here are some flavor combos that taste amazing on your favorite salad, Balance Bowl, or any other dish that needs that extra "something!"

Asian: ginger + miso + tamari + orange

Curry: coconut milk + curry powder/paste + maple syrup

Thai: coconut aminos + peanut butter + lime

Pesto: avocado + basil + garlic

Tropical: hemp + mango + lime

Cheezy: cashew + nutritional yeast + salt

Italian: sunflower seeds + sun-dried tomato + garlic + basil

Sweet: carrot + pineapple + ginger

Steps
Simply add ingredients in desired amounts to a mini blender and blend until smooth. If ingredients only require whisking, add to a small dish and use a fork to combine. Add to salad in desired amount and store extra for 2-3 days in an airtight container in the refrigerator!

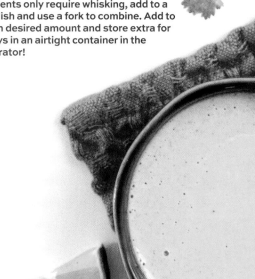

Avocados: Unripe, Too Ripe, Just Right!

When selecting an avocado at the grocery store, you want to pick one that is barely soft when you apply pressure and super dark green in color. Many times the store will only have hard green avocados in stock. Then you simply need to let them sit out on your countertop for a day or two, or to speed up ripening, place them in a paper bag with an apple or a tomato and close it up. Both of these fruits give off a high amount of ethylene gas that will cause the avocado to ripen quickly. You can also use this trick to ripen bananas! One more tip: If the stem of the avocado "pops" off easily, then it's good to go! We tend to buy some ripe and some unripe, to stagger the ripening process. If we have too many ripe at once, we place them in the refrigerator, which will halt the ripening process.

Mason Jar Hummus Dressing

Take the guesswork (and elbow grease) out of making a salad dressing by using your favorite homemade or store-bought hummus as the base. And no blender necessary! Simply add the ingredients to a mason jar and shake! This is the ideal way to add creaminess, nutrition, and flavor to your next salad or Balance Bowl (page 119) in just a few minutes. Get creative! What additional ingredients could you shake into your hummus dressing?!

(DIY) | SERVES 2 TO 3 | TIME: 3 MINUTES

½ cup favorite store-bought hummus or Homestyle Hummus (page 213)

Sea salt and freshly ground black pepper to taste

Flavor Add-Ins (add 1 to 2; optional)

1 tablespoon Dijon mustard
1 tablespoon coconut aminos
1 tablespoon maple syrup
1 tablespoon tamari or liquid aminos
Juice of ½ lemon

½ teaspoon curry powder
1 tablespoon nutritional yeast
Onion powder to taste
Garlic powder to taste

To a mason jar, add 2 tablespoons filtered water and the hummus, salt, pepper, and choice of flavor add-ins. Screw on the lid and shake vigorously until well combined. If the hummus is too thick, add up to 2 additional tablespoons filtered water. Screw the lid back on and shake again. Drizzle over a salad or store in the refrigerator for up to 5 days.

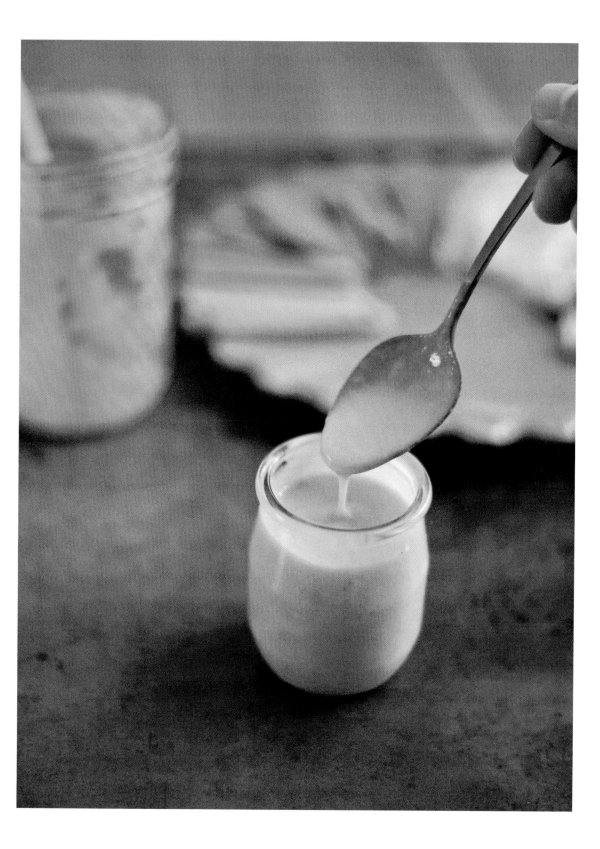

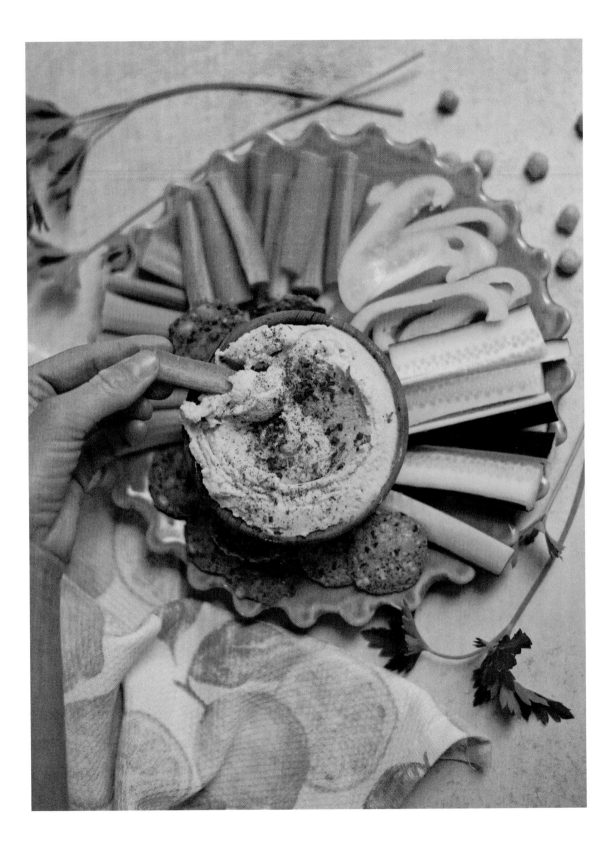

Homestyle Hummus

This easy, five-minute hummus recipe is one of our go-to snacks at home and works well paired with fresh cut veggies for dipping, spread on top of toast, dolloped on baked potatoes, or mixed into a salad. Tahini is a great source of healthy fats, chickpeas are loaded with protein, and both are rich in iron.

(K) | MAKES 2 CUPS | TIME: 5 MINUTES

1 (15.5-ounce) can chickpeas, drained and rinsed
2½ tablespoons raw tahini
½ teaspoon garlic powder
Juice of ½ lemon
¼ teaspoon ground cumin

½ teaspoon sea salt
⅛ teaspoon paprika
Freshly ground black pepper to taste
½ teaspoon curry powder (optional)
Fresh or dried parsley, for garnish

Place ¼ cup filtered water and the chickpeas, tahini, garlic powder, lemon juice, cumin, salt, paprika, pepper, and curry powder (if using) into a high-speed blender or food processor and blend until smooth. Add more water as needed to get the consistency you desire. Season with more spices or salt as needed. Garnish with the parsley. Keeps well in the refrigerator for up to 5 days.

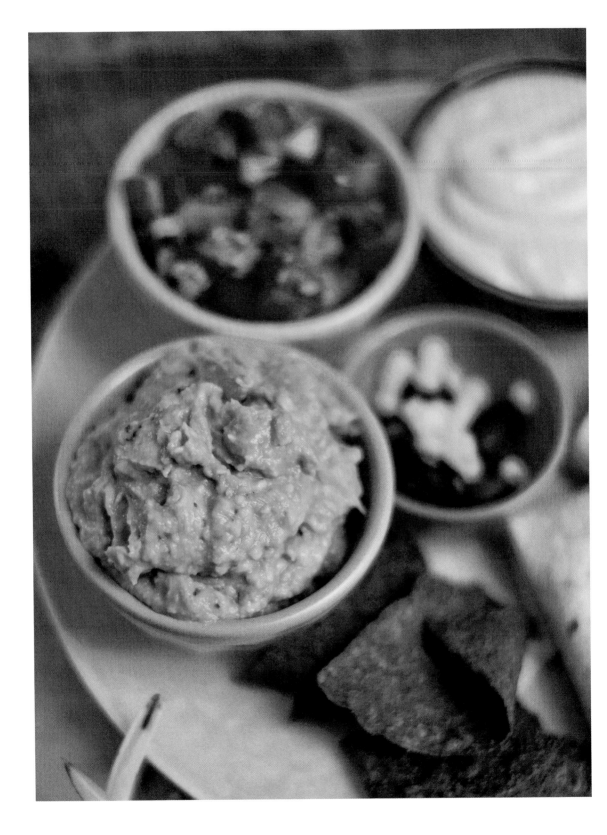

Grateful Green Guacamole

Nothing beats a perfectly ripe avocado . . . especially when mashed into a delicious guacamole! Barley grass–juice powder and/or finely chopped kale is optional, but they will enhance the nutrition of your guac without noticeably altering the taste!

(R) | SERVES 4 TO 6 | TIME: 5 MINUTES

2 or 3 ripe avocados, pitted

Juice of ½ lime

1 tablespoon chopped fresh cilantro or a few pinches of dried cilantro

1 teaspoon to 1 tablespoon barley grass–juice powder (optional)

Sea salt and freshly ground black pepper to taste

Dash of red pepper flakes or cayenne pepper

Add-ins: diced onion, minced garlic, chopped tomato, finely chopped kale (optional)

1. Scoop out the avocado flesh and discard the skin.
2. In a medium bowl, add the avocado and mash with a fork. Add the lime juice, cilantro, barley grass–juice powder (if using), salt, pepper, red pepper flakes, and your choice of add-ins and whip with a fork until well combined.
3. Dip, spread, or add a dollop to your favorite dish. Best enjoyed immediately or see the Note below regarding storage.

Note: For a lower-fat option: Thin out the fat content and add volume to the guac by blending the ingredients in a food processor with ½ medium zucchini, peeled.

To store: We've found the best way to store leftover guacamole is to put it in an airtight container and cover it with a piece of plastic wrap that is pressed down directly on top of it to reduce any exposure to air. (The citrus from the lime also helps to preserve it.) Place it in the refrigerator and eat within 24 hours.

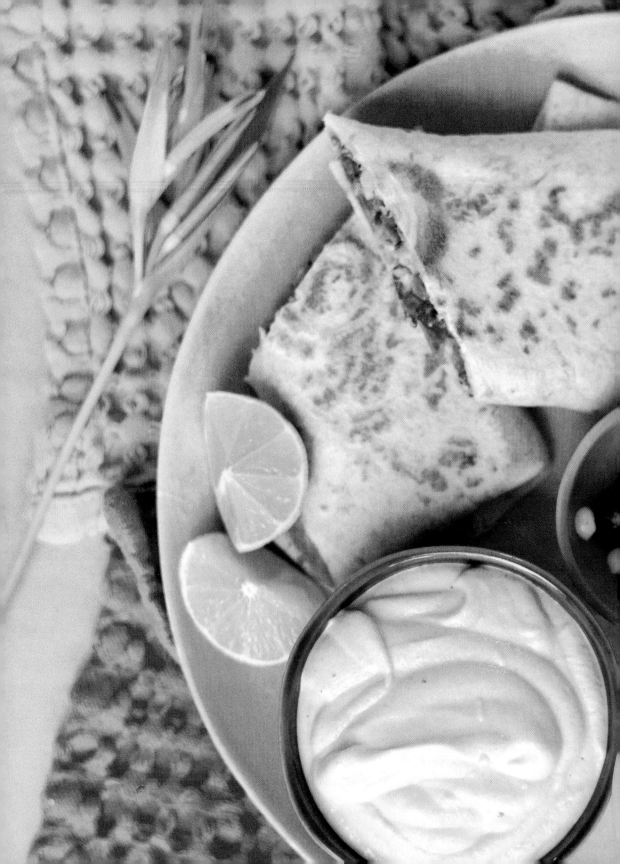

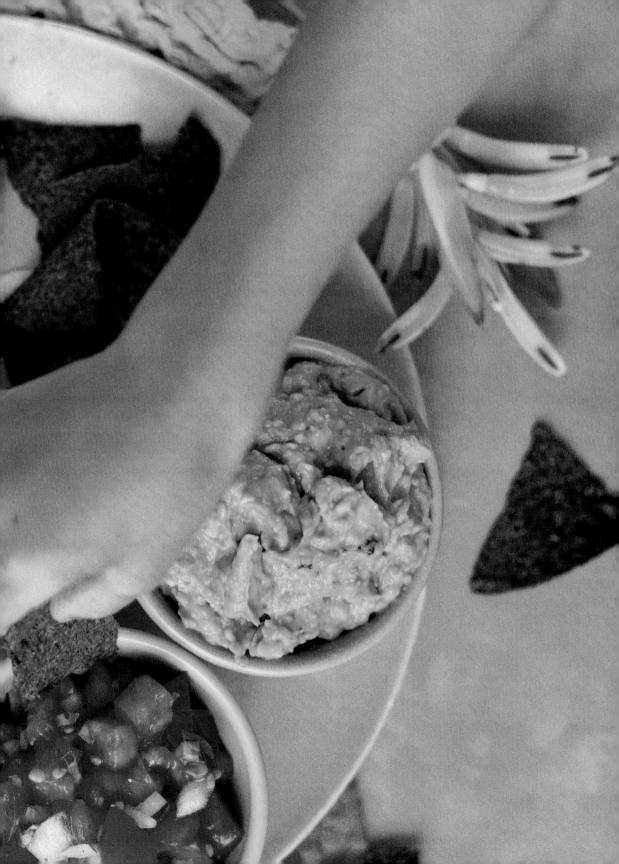

Perfect Pico de Gallo

Chunky, fresh, and flavorful, this pico de gallo is delicious eaten by the spoonful; added to tacos, nachos, or Balance Bowls (page 119); or served alongside our Grateful Green Guacamole (page 215) and Creamy Cashew Cheeze (page 219) on a burrito or wrap. For the best results, use fresh, seasonal tomatoes from your garden or farmers market.

(R) | SERVES 4 TO 6 | TIME: 5 MINUTES

4 to 5 medium tomatoes, chopped
½ red or yellow onion, chopped
2 garlic cloves, chopped
Juice of 1 lime

Handful of fresh cilantro leaves, chopped
Sea salt and freshly ground black pepper to taste
½ cup fresh mango, diced (optional, for a fruity, tropical twist!)

In a large bowl, combine the tomatoes, onion, garlic, lime juice, cilantro, salt, pepper, and mango (if using). The pico keeps well in the refrigerator for up to 5 days.

Note: For a smoother consistency, add the ingredients to a food processor and pulse to the desired texture.

Creamy Cashew Cheeze

This versatile, cheezy sauce is delicious as a dip for sweet potato fries, as a spread on your fave sandwich, spooned onto a Balance Bowl (page 119), or drizzled onto nachos. It's also easy to make and easy to digest!

(R) | MAKES 2 CUPS | TIME: 5 MINUTES

1 cup raw cashews, soaked in warm water for 4 hours or at least 30 minutes, drained and rinsed

¼ cup nutritional yeast

½ teaspoon ground turmeric

Sea salt and freshly ground black pepper to taste

Dash of garlic powder

Place the cashews, nutritional yeast, turmeric, salt, pepper, and garlic powder as well as a splash of filtered water into a high-speed blender or food processor and blend until smooth and creamy! Add more water as needed to get to your desired consistency. Dip it, slather it, drizzle it, or spread it! Store the cheeze in an airtight container in the refrigerator for up to 5 days.

Variations: Blend ½ red bell pepper into the sauce to achieve a more vibrant yellow-orange color. For a queso blanco (white) cheeze, omit the turmeric. For some extra flavor, try adding a ½ teaspoon ground cumin and a pinch of chili powder.

Colorful Salad Dressing Trio

Sweet Sunshine Salad Dressing

Bold, bright, zesty, sweet, and slightly spicy, this dressing is best enjoyed on an Asian-inspired salad or over ingredients such as green-leaf lettuce, purple cabbage, green onion, carrots, bell peppers, daikon radishes, and shiitake mushrooms. Ginger and pineapple are fantastic at fighting inflammation, and this dressing also boasts a healthy dose of vitamins A and C. Because it's fat-free, you may opt to include a sprinkle of nuts, such as slivered almonds or walnuts, or seeds to your salad.

(R) | SERVES 1 | TIME: 5 MINUTES

2 carrots, peeled and chopped
½ cup fresh pineapple, chopped

1 teaspoon minced fresh ginger

Place the carrots, pineapple, and ginger into a high-speed blender and blend until smooth.

Hot-Pink Pitaya Salad Dressing

This is my go-to when I'm craving a tangy, savory–flavored dressing! When whisked together tahini and lemon create a thick and smooth dressing that's amazing atop a fruity summer salad with kale, arugula, berries, sweet peppers, and cherry tomatoes. A touch of pitaya (dragon fruit) powder adds the perfect pop of tropical color.

(R) | SERVES 1 | TIME: 5 MINUTES

2 tablespoons raw tahini
Juice of 1 lemon

1 teaspoon pitaya powder

In a small bowl, whisk together the tahini, lemon juice, and pitaya powder until smooth. Add a touch of filtered water if the dressing becomes too thick for your liking.

> **Note:** Omit pitaya for a dressing that is great drizzled on top of white potatoes or sweet potatoes. Add a small chunk of raw red beet or beetroot powder to get the pop of pink color. If using raw beet, combine ingredients in a blender.

Tropical Mango Salad Dressing

This dressing is sweet, creamy, and smooth, and it's full of omega-3 fatty acids, protein, iron, and vitamins A and C. Try drizzling this blend over our Fiesta Color Wheel Salad (page 123) or as a dip for fresh sliced fruit.

(R) | SERVES 2 | TIME: 5 MINUTES

1 fresh ripe, juicy mango, cut into chunks or 1½ cups frozen mango chunks, thawed

Juice of 1½ limes
2 tablespoons hemp seeds

Place the mango, lime juice, and hemp seeds into a high-speed blender and blend until smooth.

Note: Double or triple any of these dressing recipes and store in an airtight container in the refrigerator for up to 3 days.

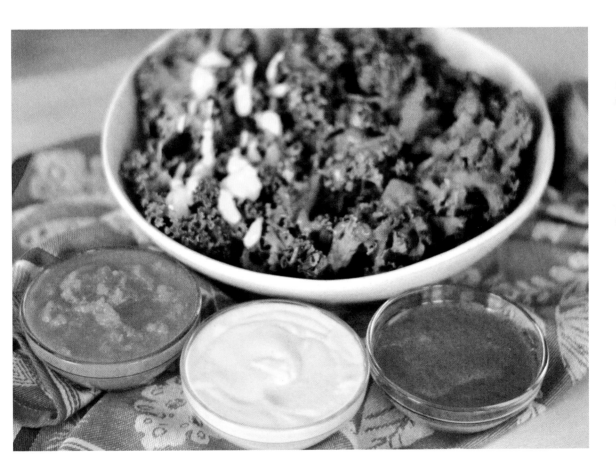

Delectable Desserts

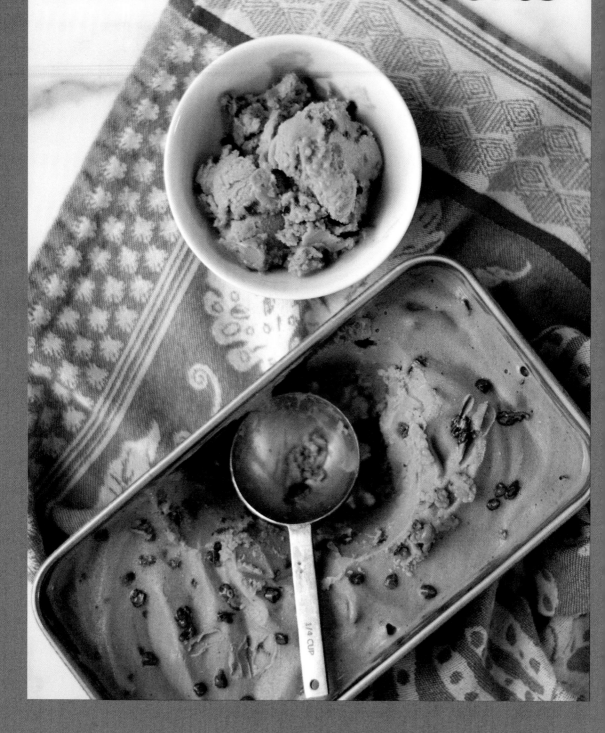

These sweet treats are sure to satisfy, and the best part is, they're all guilt-free! Try whipping up our sweet and simple Caramel Delight Cookies (page 232) or our Raw Rainbow Fruit Pizza (page 227) for a special occasion. Each of these is the perfect example of desserts not having to be the enemy.

Frothy Hot Cacao

This incredibly smooth, antioxidant-packed, superfood version of a wintertime classic will appeal to anyone—plant-based/dairy-free or not! The froth alone is enough to win over the heart of any warm beverage connoisseur, and your body will thank you for this chocolaty, not-so-guilty pleasure.

SERVES 1 | TIME: 5 MINUTES

1 cup unsweetened plant milk of choice (we like oat, soy, or almond)

1 tablespoon raw cacao powder

2 or 3 Medjool dates, pitted and soaked for at least 20 minutes in warm water

½ teaspoon vanilla bean powder or extract

1 teaspoon chocolate plant-based protein powder (optional)

Pinch of sea salt

Drop of peppermint extract or food-grade peppermint essential oil (optional)

Shredded coconut, ground cinnamon, vanilla powder, and cacao nibs, for topping (optional)

1. Add the plant milk, cacao powder, dates, vanilla, protein powder (if using), salt, and peppermint extract (if using) to a high-speed blender and blend until smooth.
2. Pour the liquid into a small saucepan and warm over low heat until the desired temperature is reached.
3. Fill up your favorite mug, sprinkle with your choice of toppings, pop in a movie, cozy up, and sip.

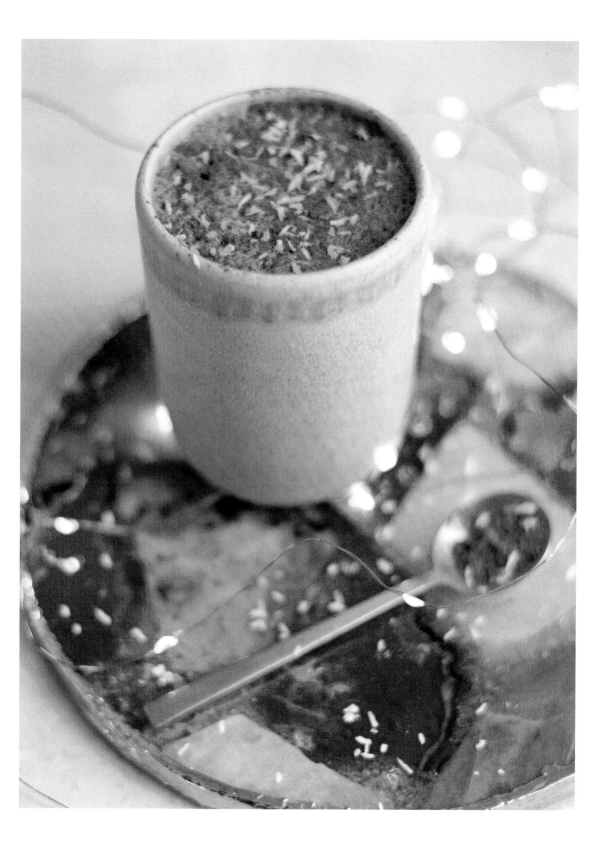

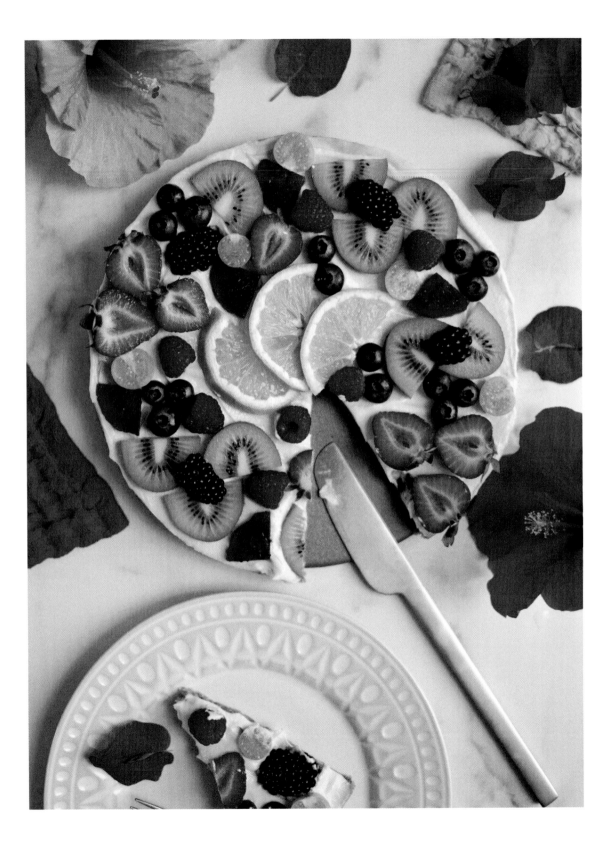

Raw Rainbow Fruit Pizza

I loved making rainbow fruit pizza with my mom growing up so I created this raw version. It's a showstopper and will wow your friends with what can be done with living foods!

(R) | SERVES 8 TO 12 | TIME: 40 MINUTES

15 to 20 Medjool dates, pitted

2 to 3 cups raw pecans, almonds, or walnuts

2 cups raw cashews, soaked in warm water for 4 hours or at least 30 minutes, drained and rinsed

2 tablespoons maple syrup or agave nectar

1 teaspoon lemon zest

3 tablespoons fresh lemon juice

Pinch of sea salt

1 teaspoon vanilla bean powder or extract

Fresh fruit of choice (berries, kiwi, mandarins)

1. In a medium bowl, add the pitted dates, cover with warm water, and soak for 20 minutes.
2. Add the pecans to a food processor and pulse into a fine meal. While the food processor is running, add a few dates at a time until the mixture is a sticky consistency.
3. Press the pecan mixture firmly into the bottom of a spring-form pan or pie tin.
4. Place ¼ cup filtered water and the cashews, maple syrup, lemon zest, lemon juice, salt, and vanilla in a high-speed blender and blend. If more water is needed to achieve a smooth, creamy consistency, add liquid slowly and continue blending until the cashews are completely blended. Spread over the pecan crust and top with fruit.
5. Place in the fridge or freezer to firm up for at least 1 hour. If frozen, remove and allow to thaw for 10 minutes, slice, and enjoy! Keeps best in an airtight container in the refrigerator for up to 3 days or in the freezer for up to 1 month.

Mint Chip Nice Cream

This dairy-free dessert can also be enjoyed for breakfast! With a base of frozen ripe bananas and the addition of any other frozen fruit or superfoods you like, you can create a delicious, dairy-free delight. We like to call it nice cream because it loves you back! Mint chip is one of our favorite classic flavors.

(R) (DIY) | SERVES 2 TO 4 | TIME: 10 MINUTES

6 frozen ripe bananas (thawed for a few minutes before blending so the appliance will not overheat and to prevent the blades from becoming dull)

Splash of unsweetened plant milk or filtered water

1 scoop vanilla plant-based protein powder (optional)

1 teaspoon spirulina or barley grass–juice powder

1 drop food-grade peppermint essential oil or ⅛ teaspoon pure peppermint extract

⅛ to ¼ cup raw cacao nibs

1. Place the frozen bananas, plant milk, protein powder (if using), spirulina, and peppermint oil in a high-speed blender. Blend until smooth, adding more milk or water as needed, to achieve desired consistency.

2. Transfer to a large bowl, fold in the cacao nibs, and enjoy immediately, or for a firmer texture, place the mixture in a freezer-safe container and freeze for 1 hour. Remove from the freezer and allow to soften for 5 minutes. Scoop with an ice cream scoop and enjoy by itself or alongside a tasty dessert. Keeps best in an airtight container in the freezer for up to 1 month.

Note: We also love making plain vanilla or chocolate nice cream with just bananas, vanilla, or chocolate plant-based protein powder and plant milk. Get creative and try combinations like strawberry banana (sweet), mango pineapple (tropical), or bananas, berries, and passion fruit (tart).

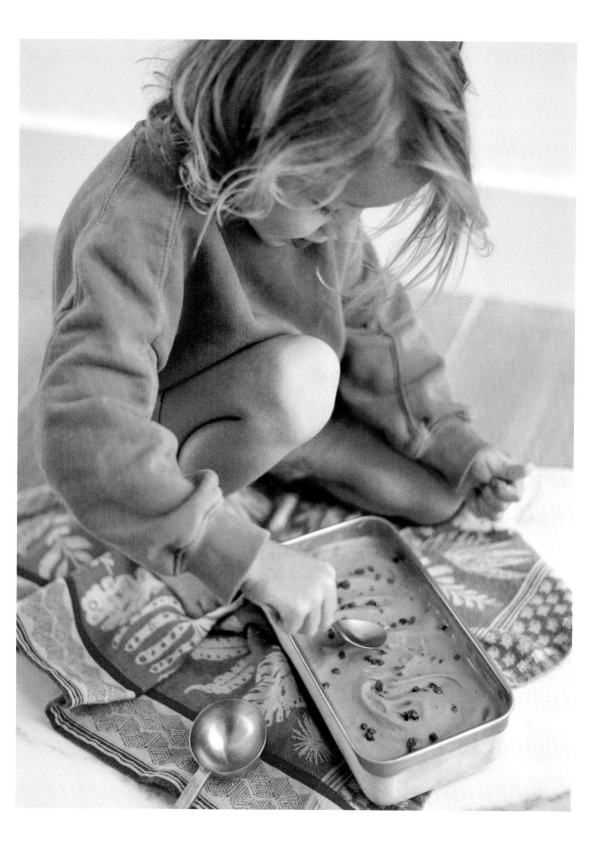

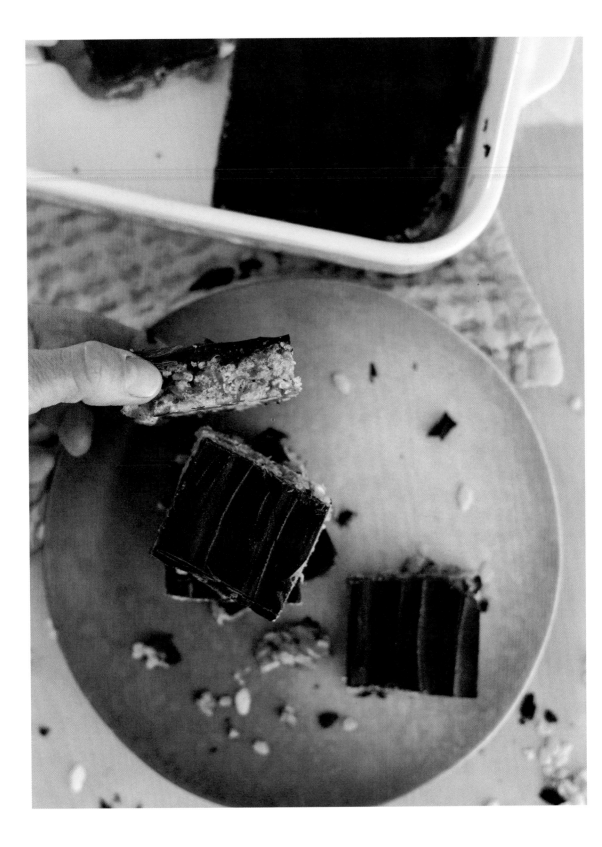

Peanut Butter Chocolate Rice Crispy Bars

Nothing beats the peanut butter and chocolate combo, and these bars are so easy because they require no baking. They are definitely a kid favorite!

(K) | MAKES 12 TO 15 BARS | TIME: 30 MINUTES

10 to 12 Medjool dates, pitted and soaked for at least 20 minutes in warm water

¾ cup peanut butter or other nut/seed butter of choice

2 teaspoons vanilla extract

Generous pinch of sea salt

3 cups unsweetened brown-rice crisps

1 (9-ounce) bag vegan dark chocolate chips

1. Add the dates, peanut butter, vanilla, and salt to a high-speed blender or food processor and blend until gooey and soft.
2. In a medium pot, warm the date mixture over medium-low heat until softened enough that you can mash and mix it with your hands.
3. In a large mixing bowl, combine the date mixture and brown-rice crisps, mixing with your hands until the crisps are evenly coated.
4. Line a 9 × 13-inch baking dish with parchment paper, pour the mixture into the dish, and evenly spread it out, pressing firmly. Place in the freezer to chill for 20 minutes.
5. In a small pot, melt the chocolate chips over medium-low heat, stirring continuously. Pour over the base and pop the dish back into the freezer to set for 30 minutes, or until the chocolate has solidified. Remove, allow to thaw for 5 minutes, cut into squares, and enjoy! These are best enjoyed right away, or stored covered in the freezer for a few weeks to avoid getting soggy.

Caramel Delight Cookies

This is one of our most popular recipes and for good reason—these cookies are to live for! They're chewy, gooey, and super fun to make with kiddos!

MAKES 12 TO 16 COOKIES | TIME: 20 MINUTES

1 cup rolled oats
10 to 12 Medjool dates, pitted and soaked for at least 20 minutes in warm water
3 tablespoons almond butter
3 tablespoons shredded coconut

1½ teaspoons vanilla bean powder or extract
Dash of sea salt
½ cup cacao paste or vegan dark chocolate chips

1. Preheat the oven to 350°F. Line a baking sheet with parchment paper.
2. In a large bowl, mash the oats, dates, almond butter, shredded coconut, vanilla, and salt together with your hands until the mixture is gooey and well combined.
3. Form 12 round balls, flatten, and place on the prepared baking sheet.
4. Bake for 10 to 12 minutes, or until the cookies just barely begin to turn golden on top, and remove from the oven.
5. In a small saucepan over low heat, melt the cacao paste, stirring often. Drizzle on top of the cookies and pop into the freezer for 25 minutes to solidify. Remove from the freezer and allow to thaw for 5 minutes and enjoy. The cookies keep best in an airtight container in the refrigerator for up to 5 days or in the freezer for up to 1 month.

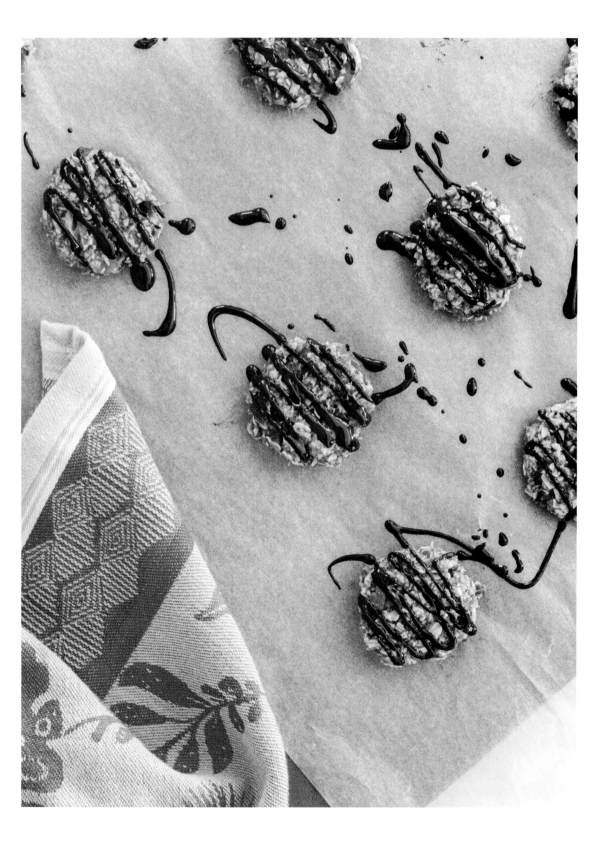

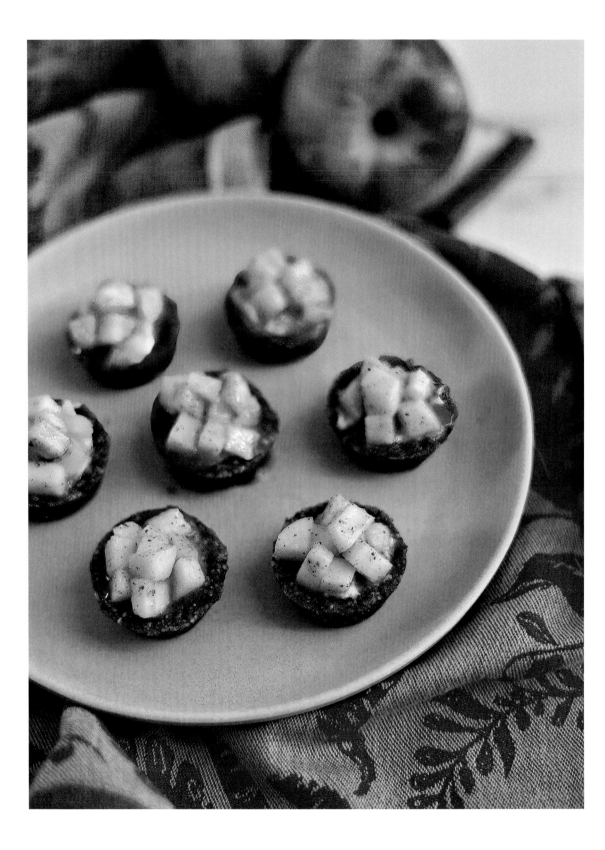

Caramel Apple Cheesecake Bites

No one will even know it's not real cheesecake—these are that good. This is another recipe sure to wow someone with just how delicious raw, living foods really can be!

(R) | MAKES 10 TO 12 BITES | TIME: 45 MINUTES

1 cup raw almonds

⅔ cup dried white mulberries or raisins

2 tablespoons ground flaxseeds

2 cups cored, peeled, and diced Granny Smith or Honeycrisp apples

1 cup raw cashews, soaked in warm water for 4 hours or at least 30 minutes, drained and rinsed

3 tablespoons maple syrup

½ teaspoon lemon juice

½ teaspoon vanilla extract

1½ tablespoons raw almond butter

Pinch of sea salt

1. In a food processor, grind the almonds into a fine meal. Add the mulberries and flaxseeds and continue grinding into a fine flour. Add 4 tablespoons filtered water and pulse until the dough holds together. You may need to add more water to reach the desired consistency. Press the dough into mini cupcake or tart pans, and place in the freezer to set for 15 minutes.
2. Place 1 cup of the apples, the cashews, 1 tablespoon of the maple syrup, the lemon juice, and ¼ teaspoon of the vanilla extract into a high-speed blender and blend until smooth. Spoon the apple cheesecake mixture onto the base and place back in the freezer to set for 30 minutes.
3. In a small bowl, whisk together the remaining 2 tablespoons maple syrup, the remaining ¼ teaspoon vanilla extract, the almond butter, and the salt. Fold in the remaining 1 cup apples until evenly coated. Spoon a bit into each cheesecake tart and enjoy! You can pop the bites into the freezer or refrigerator to firm them up and store in an airtight container in the freezer for up to a few weeks.

Note: Lining the cupcake pans with parchment paper or using silicone cupcake pans makes it easier to remove the bites.

Classic Carrot Cake

Another fan favorite over here, this spring-y recipe is made with ingredients that could classify it as a breakfast, but it tastes like a dessert, and that means, yup, you guessed it—you can eat this one whenever you like!

SERVES 12 | TIME: 90 MINUTES

Cake

1¾ cups rolled oats
2 teaspoons ground cinnamon
1 teaspoon vanilla bean powder or extract
½ teaspoon ground nutmeg
Pinch of ground cloves
2 teaspoons baking powder
1 teaspoon baking soda

10 Medjool dates, pitted and soaked for at least 20 minutes in warm water
1 fresh ripe banana
1½ cups unsweetened plant milk
3 carrots, peeled and finely grated
½ cup raw walnuts, chopped

Vanilla Cream Frosting

6 to 8 Medjool dates, pitted and soaked for at least 20 minutes in warm water
¾ cup raw cashews, soaked for at least 30 minutes and drained

1 teaspoon vanilla bean powder or extract
Juice of ½ lemon (optional, for a cream cheese flavor)

1. Preheat the oven to 350°F.
2. Place the oats in a high-speed blender and blend into a fine flour.
3. In a large mixing bowl, combine the oat flour, cinnamon, vanilla, nutmeg, cloves, baking powder, and baking soda and mix well.
4. Place the dates, banana, and plant milk in a high-speed blender and blend until smooth.
5. Add the date mixture, shredded carrots, and chopped walnuts to the dry ingredients and mix until well combined.
6. Line a 9-inch square baking dish with parchment paper, pour in the batter, and bake for 40 to 50 minutes, or the until the top is golden brown and a toothpick inserted into the center comes out clean.
7. Remove from the oven and allow to cool for 10 to 15 minutes.
8. To make the frosting, place the dates, cashews, vanilla, and lemon juice as well as just enough water to cover into a high-speed blender and blend until smooth. Spread over the cooled cake and enjoy! Keeps best in an airtight container in the refrigerator for up to 3 days.

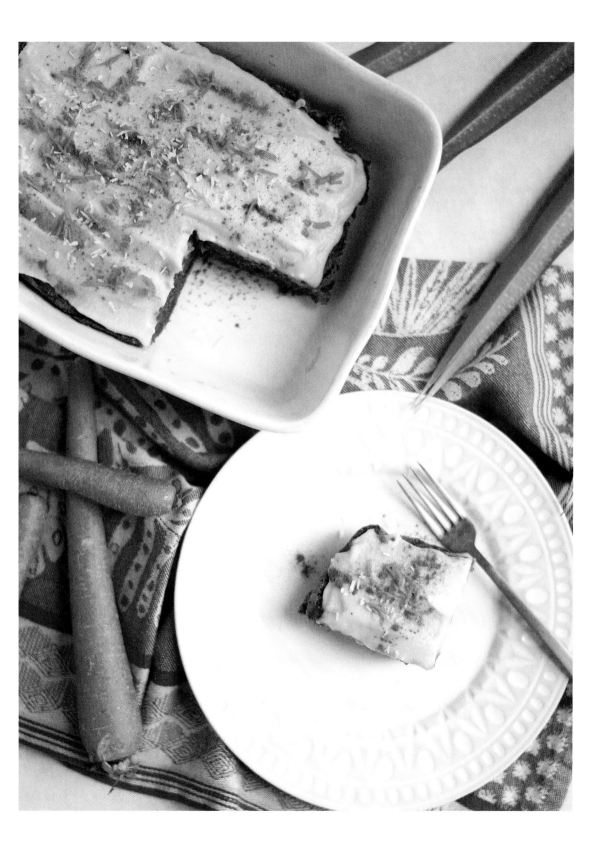

A Bright Future

We want to thank you so much for journeying through this book with us. Hopefully you've got some new favorite plant-powered recipes to add to your rotation and a better handle on the basics. There is so much in this world that is out of our control, so let's hold one another accountable to take control of what we can! With every bite, with every step, with every sleep, continue to ask yourself, are my habits helping me or hindering me?

Give yourself a pat on the back for keeping an open mind and a willing heart on this approach to a new way of doing life. Not only are you setting up yourself for success, you're setting up future generations as well. Eating more plants is amazing for our health, but it's also better for the planet and the animals that inhabit it. It's a win-win-win, and you're a part of that movement just by leaning into a plant-based diet.

We know how difficult it can be to stay the course, especially if friends and family aren't on board, but we've found through experience, that the longer we've stuck to our guns and led by example, the more people we've brought with us.

This lifestyle is so abundant, and we want you to embrace that. No more restriction, no more deprivation—find food freedom by allowing yourself to enjoy the variety of colorful foods available to you that will love you back! We also want to encourage you to place your focus on building your body up rather than breaking it down when it comes to fitness. When we focus on building strength, losing weight will take care of itself. And remember, rest does not equal laziness. There is a time and place to hustle hard, but when we rest, we repair, and when we repair, we grow!

The future is bright! Get back to the basics and Eat Move Rest Your Best with a brand new mindset—abundance, light, color, empowerment, freedom, strength, and positivity.

Sending you so much love and support,
Erin and Dusty

What's Next

Join our email list at EatMoveRest.com to instantly receive a free seven-day video guide addressing a different area of concern each day, from weight loss to hormonal health to building lean muscle.

If you're hungry for more, be sure to check out the Eat Move Rest Club! Our online membership program houses all our digital content plus a thriving community of like-mined individuals.

Eat Move Rest Club member perks

Meal planner and recipe app
   (also includes workouts, meditations, and wellness articles)
Recipe ebooks and getting-started PDFs
Private Facebook community
Weekly livestream Q & A videos
Monthly group Zoom coaching w/ occasional guest experts
Accountability and connection to reach your health goals
. . . and so much more!

Connect with us!

Be sure to join in the online community and Eat Move Rest Your Best with us on social media!
Our social media channels:

Website: EatMoveRest.com
Membership: Membership.EatMoveRest.com
Product faves and discount codes: EatMoveRest.com/Our-Faves
YouTube: @EatMoveRest
Instagram: @ErinStanczyk @DBStanczyk @EatMoveRest
Facebook: @EatMoveRest
TikTok: @EatMoveRest

Be sure to tag us @EatMoveRest and #EatMoveRest to show us how you do it!

Acknowledgments

First and foremost, we want to thank our family, friends, and the Eat Move Rest community. Your continual support and encouragement inspires us daily.

We also want to give so much love to our sweet little ones, Max, Liv, and Zoe and our big furry baby, Beau—you're the best taste-testers around!

Dusty and I are also thankful for each other. We could not have created any of this without our divide-and-conquer teamwork and picking each other up when we had our doubts. From recipe development and prep to food styling and photography, we pat ourselves on the back for tackling this massive undertaking as a couple and distilling our years of Eat Move Rest philosophy into a streamlined guide for our readers.

Thank you to our parents who taught us how to work hard and continually encouraged us to pursue our passions with the reminder that we could do anything we put our minds to.

Thank you to our publishing team at HarperCollins, including our super supportive editors Sydney Rogers, Katy Hamilton, Maya Alpert, and Julia Pastore. A special thanks to our agent, the late Bill Gladstone, for believing in us and our vision.

Thank you to photographers Devon Stanczyk, Ariel Panowicz, and Miranda Rossi for capturing such special photos of our family in this book and over the years.

Thank you to our mentor and fellow author friend, Joel Christiansen, who taught us to keep a can-do attitude and reminded us "you can't fail with detail."

Thank you to our friends and family members who provided us feedback in exchange for meals and encouraged us through the book-writing process.

Finally, we want to thank YOU, the reader, for picking up this book. We hope and pray you found a little slice of heaven within, and that you will treasure what you've learned and the recipes you've created for years to come!

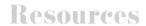

Resources

General plant-based nutrition books, documentaries, websites, podcasts, and other resources:

Some of our favorite physicians, specialists, and experts in the field:

Will Bulsiewicz, MD, gastroenterologist, author of *Fiber Fueled*

Caldwell B. Esselstyn, MD, cardiologist, author of *Prevent and Reverse Heart Disease*

Brooke Goldner, MD, author of *Goodbye Lupus* and *Goodbye Autoimmune Disease*

Michael Greger, MD, founder of NutritionFacts.org and author of *How Not to Die*

Simon Hill, RD, creator of *The Proof Podcast* and author of *The Proof Is in the Plants*

Michael Klaper, MD, author of *Vegan Nutrition: Pure and Simple*

Gemma Newman, MD, pediatrician, obstetrician, and gynecologist, author of *The Plant Power Doctor*

Dean Ornish, MD, internal medicine, author of *Undo It!: How Simple Lifestyle Changes Can Reverse Most Chronic Diseases*

Rich Roll, ultra-athlete, creator of *The Rich Roll Podcast* and author of *Finding Ultra*

Dean Sherzai, MD, PhD, and Ayesha Sherzai, MD, neuroscientists, authors of *The Alzheimer's Solution*

Books:

Buettner, Dan. *The Blue Zones*. Washington, DC: National Geographic Society, 2008.

Campbell, T. Colin. *Whole*. Dallas: BenBella Books: 2013.

Campbell, T. Colin, and Thomas M. Campbell II, MD. *The China Study*. Dallas: BenBella Books, 2016.

Davis, Brenda, and Vesanto Melina. *Becoming Vegan*. Summertown, TN: Book Publishing Company, 2000.

Graham, Douglas N. *The 80/10/10 Diet*. St. Petersburg, FL: FoodnSport Press, 2006.

Greger, Michael. *How Not to Die*. New York: Flatiron Books, 2015.

Lisle, Douglas J., and Alan Goldhamer. *The Pleasure Trap*. Summertown, TN: Healthy Living Publications, 2003.

Documentaries:

Andersen, Kip, and Keegan Kuhn, dirs. *Cowspiracy*. 2014, Netflix.

Andersen, Kip, and Keegan Kuhm, dirs. *What the Health*. 2017, Netflix.

Fulkerson, Lee. *Forks Over Knives*. 2011, Virgil Films and Entertainment.

Reference websites and publications:

Evidence-Based Eating Guide (https://nutritionfacts.org/healthkit/), Michael Greger, MD

Forks Over Knives magazine

International Journal of Disease Reversal and Prevention

NutritionFacts.org, Michael Greger, MD

YouTube:

Graham, Douglas. "Humans vs. Carnivores." YouTube, https://youtu.be/c7e_Ye6Yu6I?si=N6BXnIosw0FcccUL.

Podcasts:

Hill, Simon. *The Proof Podcast*

Roll, Rich. *The Rich Roll Podcast*

Plant-based pregnancy, baby, and child resources to explore:

Guide: Pediatric Plant-Based Nutrition Quick Start Guide (www.plantricianproject.org/quickstartguide), a super helpful short read to ensure you and your baby or child are getting what you need

Website: Physicians Committee for Responsible Medicine (https://www.pcrm.org), includes guidance specific to vegan pregnancies

Physician: Gemma Newman, MD, pediatrician, obstetrician, and gynecologist, author of *The Plant Power Doctor*

Dieticians: Whitney English and Alexandra Caspero, Plant-Based Juniors (www.plantbasedjuniors.com), a great website, IG account, and book, *The Plant-Based Baby and Toddler*, filled with lots of recipes and information on supplementation and nutrition

Books: *The Kind Mama* by Alicia Silverstone, on vegan pregnancy and childbirth, and *Your Complete Vegan Pregnancy* by Reed Mangels, on proper nutrition for all three trimesters

Kitchen tools, products, and supplements with discount codes to explore:

EatMoveRest.com/our-faves

Universal Conversion Chart

Oven Temperature Equivalents

250°F =	120°C	400°F =	200°C
275°F –	135°C	425°F =	220°C
300°F =	150°C	450°F =	230°C
325°F =	160°C	475°F =	240°C
350°F =	180°C	500°F =	260°C
375°F =	190°C		

Measurement Equivalents

Measurements should always be level unless directed otherwise.

⅛ teaspoon = 0.5 mL

¼ teaspoon = 1 mL

½ teaspoon = 2.5 mL

1 teaspoon = 5 mL

1 tablespoon = 3 teaspoons = ½ fluid ounce = 15 mL

2 tablespoons = ⅛ cup = 1 fluid ounce = 30 mL

4 tablespoons = ¼ cup = 2 fluid ounces = 60 mL

5⅓ tablespoons = ⅓ cup = 3 fluid ounces = 80 mL

8 tablespoons = ½ cup = 4 fluid ounces = 120 mL

10⅔ tablespoons = ⅔ cup = 5 fluid ounces = 160 mL

12 tablespoons = ¾ cup = 6 fluid ounces = 180 mL

16 tablespoons = 1 cup = 8 fluid ounces = 240 mL

Index

NOTE: Page references in *italics* indicate photos of recipes.

About the Authors

Erin and Dusty Stanczyk were both born and raised in the Midwest and connected after college. Erin had received her degree in biological sciences and Dusty, communication studies. The two combined forces, and with Erin's science-minded approach to nutrition and Dusty's interpersonal skills, they embarked upon a training program to become certified health and lifestyle coaches. Meanwhile, the two were on a quest to uncover the root cause of their own individual health struggles already weighing on them in their twenties.

While attending conferences and doing their own research, the two continued to find more and more evidence supporting the power of a plant-based diet and using food as medicine. After giving it a go for forty days, they were convinced! The longer they stuck with their new lifestyle—not just eating better but moving daily and getting quality rest—the better they felt, and it became woven into every conversation they had.

Eventually, they created EatMoveRest.com as a hub to house all their findings, from sharing their favorite green smoothie and other delicious plant-based recipes to reporting the facts and sharing helpful resources. As their knowledge and experience grew, so did their social media presence and online community. Their YouTube channel took off, and before they knew it, they were rounding up friends and followers from all across the world to join them on healing retreats in Costa Rica.

Amid the success of their budding business, they also became a plant-based family of three, and then four, and now five! When they're not juicing, blending, and chopping in the kitchen, Erin, Dusty, Max, Liv, Zoe, and their Bernese mountain dog, Beau, enjoy spending time outside and staying active. They travel and explore as much as possible, and they enjoy connecting with their Eat Move Rest community both online and in person. They've got big plans to spread their message and philosophy to all the ends of the Earth, in hopes to cultivate better health and harmony for all living beings.

Be sure to follow and connect with Erin and Dusty on Instagram @EriStanczyk and @DBStanczyk as well as @EatMoveRest on YouTube, Instagram, Facebook, and TikTok! Sign up for the Eat Move Rest email list to get a free seven-day video guide to living your best and healthiest life and join the Eat Move Rest Club online community.